Pediatrics, Child and Adolescent Health

Bicycles

Helmet Use of Adolescents at Independent Schools

PEDIATRICS, CHILD AND ADOLESCENT HEALTH

JOAV MERRICK - SERIES EDITOR
NATIONAL INSTITUTE OF CHILD HEALTH
AND HUMAN DEVELOPMENT,
MINISTRY OF SOCIAL AFFAIRS, JERUSALEM

Bicycles: Helmet Use of Adolescents at Independent Schools
Ronald Chow, Michael Borean, Drew Hollenberg, Jaclyn Viehweger, Tharani Anpalagan and Anna Rzepka (Editors)
2017. ISBN: 978-1-53612-458-3 (Softcover)
2017. ISBN: 978-1-53612-459-0 (e-book)

Positive Youth Development: Long Term Effects in a Chinese Program
Daniel TL Shek, Cecilia MS Ma, Janet TY Leung and Joav Merrick (Editors)
2017. ISBN: 978-1-53612-539-9 (Hardcover)
2017. ISBN: 978-1-53612-540-5 (e-book)

Adolescence: Bicycle and Helmet Use of Adolescents and Young Adults
Ronald Chow and Joav Merrick (Editors)
2017. ISBN: 978-1-53612-039-4 (Hardcover)
2017. ISBN: 978-1-53612-060-8 (e-book)

Suicide: A Global View on Suicidal Ideation among Adolescents
Mazyanga L. Mazaba, Seter Siziya and Joav Merrick (Editors)
2017. ISBN: 978-1-53611-788-2 (Hardcover)
2017. ISBN: 978-1-53611-799-8 (e-book)

Children and Youth: Post-Traumatic Stress Disorder and Motor Vehicle Crashes
Donald E. Greydanus, Roger W. Apple, Kathryn White, and Joav Merrick (Editors)
2017. ISBN: 978-1-53611-102-6 (Hardcover)
2017. ISBN: 978-1-53611-255-9 (e-book)

Child and Adolescent Health Yearbook 2016
Joav Merrick (Editor)
2017. ISBN: 978-1-53610-948-1 (Hardcover)
2017. ISBN: 978-1-53610-957-3 (e-book)

Child Health and Human Development Yearbook 2016
Joav Merrick (Editor)
2017. ISBN: 978-1-53610-946-7 (Hardcover)
2017. ISBN: 978-1-53610-958-0 (e-book)

Chronic Disease and Disability: The Pediatric Kidney
Donald E Greydanus, Vimal Master Sankar Raj, and Joav Merrick (Editors)
2016. ISBN: 978-1-63483-793-4 (Hardcover)
2015. ISBN: 978-1-63483-809-2 (e-book)

Child and Adolescent Health Yearbook 2015
Joav Merrick (Editor)
2016. ISBN: 978-1-63484-512-0 (Hardcover)
2016. ISBN: 978-1-63484-543-4 (e-book)

Child Health and Human Development Yearbook 2015
Joav Merrick (Editor)
2016. ISBN: 978-1-63484-513-7 (Hardcover)
2016. ISBN: 978-1-63484-544-1 (e-book)

Pain Management Yearbook 2015
Joav Merrick (Editor)
2016. ISBN: 978-1-63484-515-1 (Hardcover)
2016. ISBN: 978-1-63484-545-8 (e-book)

**Children and Childhood:
Some International Aspects**
Joav Merrick (Editor)
2016. ISBN: 978-1-63484-587-8
(Hardcover)
2016. ISBN: 978-1-63484-594-6
(e-book)

**Children and Adolescents:
Future Challenges**
*Daniel TL Shek, Tak Yan Lee,
and Joav Merrick (Editors)*
2016. ISBN: 978-1-63484-616-5
(Hardcover)
2016. ISBN: 978-1-63484-627-1
(e-book)

**Adolescence: Positive Youth
Development Programs
in Chinese Communities**
*Daniel TL Shek, Florence KY Wu,
Janet TY Leung, and Joav Merrick
(Editors)*
2016. ISBN: 978-1-63484-044-6
(Hardcover)
2016. ISBN: 978-1-63484-677-6
(e-book)

**Sexuality:
Some International Aspects**
*Joav Merrick
and Donald E Greydanus (Editors)*
2016. ISBN: 978-1-63484-707-0
(Hardcover)
2016. ISBN: 978-1-63484-719-3
(e-book)

**Growing Up in the Middle East:
The Daily Lives and Well-Being
of Israeli and Palestinian Youth**
*Yossi Harel-Fisch, Ziad Abdeen
and Miriam Navot*
2016. ISBN: 978-1-63484-746-9
(Hardcover)
2016. ISBN: 978-1-63484-765-0
(e-book)

**Chronic Disease and Disability:
The Pediatric Heart**
*Donald E Greydanus,
Devika Malhotra
and Joav Merrick (Editors)*
2016. ISBN: 978-1-63484-828-2
(Hardcover)
2016. ISBN: 978-1-63484-842-8
(e-book)

Diabetes Mellitus: Childhood and Adolescence
Manmohan K Kamboj, Donald E Greydanus and Joav Merrick (Editors)
2016. ISBN: 978-1-53610-095-2 (Hardcover)
2016. ISBN: 978-1-53610-104-1 (e-book)

Chronic Disease and Disability: Abuse and Neglect in Childhood and Adolescence
Donald E Greydanus, Vincent J Palusci and Joav Merrick (Editors)
2016. ISBN: 978-1-53610-129-4 (Hardcover)
2016. ISBN: 978-1-53610-142-3 (e-book)

Clinical Aspects of Psychopharmacology in Childhood and Adolescence, Second Edition
Donald E Greydanus, Joseph L Calles, Jr, Dilip R Patel, Ahsan Nazeer and Joav Merrick (Editors)
2016. ISBN: 978-1-53610-241-3 (Hardcover)
2016. ISBN: 978-1-53610-253-6 (e-book)

Chronic Disease and Disability: The Pediatric Pancreas
Donald E Greydanus, Manmohan K Kamboj and Joav Merrick (Editors)
2016. ISBN: 978-1-53610-055-6 (Hardcover)
2016. ISBN: 978-1-53610-065-5 (e-book)

A Pediatric Resident Pocket Guide: Making the Most of Morning Reports
Arthur N Feinberg
2015. ISBN: 978-1-63482-141-4 (Softcover)
2015. ISBN: 978-1-63482-186-5 (e-book)

Tropical Pediatrics: A Public Health Concern of International Proportions Second Edition
Richard R Roach, Donald E Greydanus, Dilip R Patel and Joav Merrick (Editors)
2015. ISBN: 978-1-63463-381-9 (Hardcover)
2015. ISBN: 978-1-63463-404-5 (e-book)

Child and Adolescent Health Issues (A Tribute to the Pediatrician Donald E Greydanus)
Joav Merrick (Editor)
2015. ISBN: 978-1-63463-574-5 (Hardcover)
2015. ISBN: 978-1-63463-576-9 (e-book)

Child and Adolescent Health Yearbook 2014
Joav Merrick (Editor)
2015. ISBN: 978-1-63482-162-9 (Hardcover)
2015. ISBN: 978-1-63482-206-0 (e-book)

Child Health and Human Development Yearbook 2014
Joav Merrick (Editor)
2015. ISBN: 978-1-63482-163-6 (Hardcover)
2015. ISBN: 978-1-63482-207-7 (e-book)

Behavioral Pediatrics, 4th Edition
Donald E Greydanus, Dilip R Patel, Helen D Pratt, Joseph L Calles Jr, Ahsan Nazeer and Joav Merrick (Editors)
2015. ISBN: 978-1-63483-027-0 (Hardcover)
2015. ISBN: 978-1-63483-052-2 (e-book)

Disability, Chronic Disease and Human Development
Joav Merrick
2015. ISBN: 978-1-63483-029-4 (Hardcover)
2015. ISBN: 978-1-63483-057-7 (e-book)

**Caribbean Adolescents:
Some Public Health Concerns**
*Cecilia Hegamin-Younge
and Joav Merrick (Editors)*
2015. ISBN: 978-1-63483-341-7
(Hardcover)
2015. ISBN: 978-1-63483-343-1
(e-book)

**Adolescence and Health:
Some International Perspectives**
Joav Merrick (Editor)
2015. ISBN: 978-1-63483-791-0
(Hardcover)
2015. ISBN: 978-1-63483-808-5
(e-book)

**Youth Suicide Prevention:
Everybody's Business**
Hatim A Omar (Editor)
2015. ISBN: 978-1-63483-786-6
(Softcover)
2015. ISBN: 978-1-63483-820-7
(e-book)

**Human Developmental Research:
Experience from Research
in Hong Kong**
*Daniel TL Shek, Cecilia Ma, Yu Lu
and Joav Merrick (Editors)*
2014. ISBN: 978-1-62808-166-4
(Hardcover)
2013. ISBN: 978-1-62808-167-1
(e-book)

**School, Adolescence
and Health Issues**
*Joav Merrick, Ariel Tenenbaum
and Hatim A Omar (Editors)*
2014. ISBN: 978-1-62948-702-1
(Hardcover)
2014. ISBN: 978-1-62948-707-6
(e-book)

**Adolescence and Sexuality:
International Perspectives**
*Joav Merrick, Ariel Tenenbaum
and Hatim A Omar (Editors)*
2014. ISBN: 978-1-62948-711-3
(Hardcover)
2014. ISBN: 978-1-62948-724-3
(e-book)

Child and Adolescent Health Yearbook 2013
Joav Merrick (Editor)
2014. ISBN: 978-1-63117-658-6
(Hardcover)
2014. ISBN: 978-1-63117-668-5
(e-book)

**Adoption:
The Search for a New Parenthood**
*Gary Diamond and Eva Arbel
(Israel)*
2014. ISBN: 978-1-63117-710-1
(Hardcover)
2014. ISBN: 978-1-63117-713-2
(e-book)

Adolescence: Places and Spaces
*Myra F Taylor, Julie Ann Pooley
and Joav Merrick (Editors)*
2014. ISBN: 978-1-63117-847-4
(Hardcover)
2014. ISBN: 978-1-63117-850-4
(e-book)

Pain Management Yearbook 2013
Joav Merrick (Editor)
2014. ISBN: 978-1-63117-944-0
(Hardcover)
2014. ISBN: 978-1-63117-959-4
(e-book)

Child Health and Human Development Yearbook 2013
Joav Merrick (Editor)
2014. ISBN: 978-1-63117-939-6
(Hardcover)
2013. ISBN: 978-1-63117-958-7
(e-book)

**Born into this World:
Health Issues**
*Donald E Greydanus,
Arthur N Feinberg,
and Joav Merrick (Editors)*
2014. ISBN: 978-1-63321-667-9
(Hardcover)
2014. ISBN: 978-1-63321-669-3
(e-book)

**Caring for the Newborn:
A Comprehensive Guide
for the Clinician**
*Donald E Greydanus,
Arthur N Feinberg
and Joav Merrick (Editors)*
2014. ISBN: 978-1-63321-760-7
(Hardcover)
2014. ISBN: 978-1-63321-781-2
(e-book)

**Environment and Hope:
Improving Health, Reducing AIDS
and Promoting Food Security
in the World**
*Leslie Rubin and Joav Merrick
(Editors)*
2014. ISBN: 978-1-63321-772-0
(Hardcover)
2014. ISBN: 978-1-63321-782-9
(e-book)

**Pediatric and Adolescent
Dermatology:
Some Current Issues**
*Donald E Greydanus,
Arthur N Feinberg
and Joav Merrick (Editors)*
2014. ISBN: 978-1-63321-853-6
(Hardcover)
2014. ISBN: 978-1-63321-863-5
(e-book)

**Adolescence and Behavior Issues
in a Chinese Context**
*Daniel TL Shek, Rachel CF Sun,
and Joav Merrick (Editors)*
2013. ISBN: 978-1-62618-614-9
(Hardcover)
2013. ISBN: 978-1-62618-692-7
(e-book)

**Advances in Preterm
Infant Research**
*Jing Sun, Nicholas Buys
and Joav Merrick*
2013. ISBN: 978-1-62618-696-5
(Hardcover)
2013. ISBN: 978-1-62618-775-7
(e-book)

**Child Health and Human
Development: Social, Economic
and Environmental Factors**
*Leslie Rubin and Joav Merrick
(Editors)*
2013. ISBN: 978-1-62948-166-1
(Hardcover)
2013. ISBN: 978-1-62948-169-2
(e-book)

**Children, Violence and Bullying:
International Perspectives**
*Joav Merrick, Isack Kandel
and Hatim A Omar (Editors)*
2013. ISBN: 978-1-62948-342-9
(Hardcover)
2013. ISBN: 978-1-62948-345-0
(e-book)

Chinese Adolescent Development:
Economic Disadvantages, Parents
and Intrapersonal Development
Daniel TL Shek, Rachel CF Sun
and Joav Merrick (Editors)
2013. ISBN: 978-1-62618-622-4
(Hardcover)
2013. ISBN: 978-1-62618-694-1
(e-book)

Chronic Disease and Disability
in Childhood
Joav Merrick
2013. ISBN: 978-1-62808-865-6
(Hardcover)
2013. ISBN: 978-1-62808-868-7
(e-book)

Environmental Health Disparities
in Children: Asthma, Obesity
and Food
Leslie Rubin and Joav Merrick
(Editors)
2013. ISBN: 978-1-62948-122-7
(Hardcover)
2013. ISBN: 978-1-62948-135-7
(e-book)

Environmental Health:
Home, School and Community
Leslie Rubin and Joav Merrick
(Editors)
2013. ISBN: 978-1-62948-155-5
(Hardcover)
2013. ISBN: 978-1-62948-158-6
(e-book)

Guidelines for the Healthy
Integration of the Ill Child in the
Educational System: Experience
from Israel
Yosefa Isenberg
2013. ISBN: 978-1-62808-350-7
(Hardcover)
2013. ISBN: 978-1-62808-353-8
(e-book)

Internet Addiction: A Public
Health Concern in Adolescence
Artemis Tsitsika, Mari Janikian,
Donald E Greydanus,
Hatim A Omar
and Joav Merrick (Editors)
2013. ISBN: 978-1-62618-925-6
(Hardcover)
2013. ISBN: 978-1-62618-959-1
(e-book)

Playing with Fire: Children, Adolescents and Firesetting
Hatim A. Omar, Carrie Howell Bowling and Joav Merrick (Editors)
2013. ISBN: 978-1-62948-471-6 (Softcover)
2013. ISBN: 978-1-62948-474-7 (e-book)

Promotion of Holistic Development of Young People in Hong Kong
Daniel TL Shek, Tak Yan Lee and Joav Merrick (Editors)
2013. ISBN: 978-1-62808-019-3 (Hardcover)
2013. ISBN: 978-1-62808-040-7 (e-book)

University and College Students: Health and Development Issues for the Leaders of Tomorrow
Daniel TL Shek, Rachel CF and Joav Merrick (Editors)
2013. ISBN: 978-1-62618-586-9 (Hardcover)
2013. ISBN: 978-1-62618-612-5 (e-book)

Break the Cycle of Environmental Health Disparities: Maternal and Child Health Aspects
Leslie Rubin and Joav Merrick (Editors)
2013. ISBN: 978-1-62948-107-4 (Hardcover)
2013. ISBN: 978-1-62948-133-3 (e-book)

Child and Adolescent Health Yearbook 2012
Joav Merrick (Editor)
2012. ISBN: 978-1-61942-788-4 (Hardcover)
2012. ISBN: 978-1-61942-789-1 (e-book)

Child Health and Human Development Yearbook 2011
Joav Merrick (Editor)
2012. ISBN: 978-1-61942-969-7 (Hardcover)
2012. ISBN: 978-1-61942-970-3 (e-book)

Child and Adolescent Health Yearbook 2011
Joav Merrick (Editor)
2012. ISBN: 978-1-61942-782-2 (Hardcover)
2012. ISBN: 978-1-61942-783-9 (e-book)

**Tropical Pediatrics:
A Public Health Concern of
International Proportions**
*Richard R Roach,
Donald E Greydanus,
Dilip R Patel, Douglas N Homnick
and Joav Merrick (Editors)*
2012. ISBN: 978-1-61942-831-7
(Hardcover)
2012. ISBN: 978-1-61942-840-9
(e-book)

**Child Health and Human
Development Yearbook 2012**
Joav Merrick (Editor)
2012. ISBN: 978-1-61942-978-9
(Hardcover)
2012. ISBN: 978-1-61942-979-6
(e-book)

**Developmental Issues
in Chinese Adolescents**
*Daniel TL Shek, Rachel CF Sun
and Joav Merrick (Editors)*
2012. ISBN: 978-1-62081-262-4
(Hardcover)
2012. ISBN: 978-1-62081-270-9
(e-book)

**Positive Youth Development:
Theory, Research and Application**
*Daniel TL Shek, Rachel CF Sun
and Joav Merrick (Editors)*
2012. ISBN: 978-1-62081-305-8
(Hardcover)
2012. ISBN: 978-1-62081-347-8
(e-book)

**Understanding Autism
Spectrum Disorder:
Current Research Aspects**
*Ditza A Zachor and Joav Merrick
(Editors)*
2012. ISBN: 978-1-62081-353-9
(Hardcover)
2012. ISBN: 978-1-62081-390-4
(e-book)

**Positive Youth Development: A
New School Curriculum to Tackle
Adolescent Developmental Issues**
*Hing Keung Ma, Daniel TL Shek
and Joav Merrick (Editors)*
2012. ISBN: 978-1-62081-384-3
(Hardcover)
2012. ISBN: 978-1-62081-385-0
(e-book)

Transition from Pediatric to Adult Medical Care
*David Wood, John G Reiss,
Maria E Ferris, Linda R Edwards
and Joav Merrick (Editors)*
2012. ISBN: 978-1-62081-409-3
(Hardcover)
2012. ISBN: 978-1-62081-412-3
(e-book)

PEDIATRICS, CHILD AND ADOLESCENT HEALTH

BICYCLES

HELMET USE OF ADOLESCENTS AT INDEPENDENT SCHOOLS

RONALD CHOW
MICHAEL BOREAN
DREW HOLLENBERG
JACLYN VIEHWEGER
THARANI ANPALAGAN
AND
ANNA RZEPKA
EDITORS

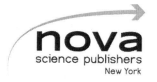

Copyright © 2017 by Nova Science Publishers, Inc.

All rights reserved. No part of this book may be reproduced, stored in a retrieval system or transmitted in any form or by any means: electronic, electrostatic, magnetic, tape, mechanical photocopying, recording or otherwise without the written permission of the Publisher.

We have partnered with Copyright Clearance Center to make it easy for you to obtain permissions to reuse content from this publication. Simply navigate to this publication's page on Nova's website and locate the "Get Permission" button below the title description. This button is linked directly to the title's permission page on copyright.com. Alternatively, you can visit copyright.com and search by title, ISBN, or ISSN.

For further questions about using the service on copyright.com, please contact:
Copyright Clearance Center
Phone: +1-(978) 750-8400   Fax: +1-(978) 750-4470   E-mail: info@copyright.com.

NOTICE TO THE READER

The Publisher has taken reasonable care in the preparation of this book, but makes no expressed or implied warranty of any kind and assumes no responsibility for any errors or omissions. No liability is assumed for incidental or consequential damages in connection with or arising out of information contained in this book. The Publisher shall not be liable for any special, consequential, or exemplary damages resulting, in whole or in part, from the readers' use of, or reliance upon, this material. Any parts of this book based on government reports are so indicated and copyright is claimed for those parts to the extent applicable to compilations of such works.

Independent verification should be sought for any data, advice or recommendations contained in this book. In addition, no responsibility is assumed by the publisher for any injury and/or damage to persons or property arising from any methods, products, instructions, ideas or otherwise contained in this publication.

This publication is designed to provide accurate and authoritative information with regard to the subject matter covered herein. It is sold with the clear understanding that the Publisher is not engaged in rendering legal or any other professional services. If legal or any other expert assistance is required, the services of a competent person should be sought. FROM A DECLARATION OF PARTICIPANTS JOINTLY ADOPTED BY A COMMITTEE OF THE AMERICAN BAR ASSOCIATION AND A COMMITTEE OF PUBLISHERS.

Additional color graphics may be available in the e-book version of this book.

Library of Congress Cataloging-in-Publication Data

ISBN: 978-1-53612-458-3

Published by Nova Science Publishers, Inc. † New York

CONTENTS

Section one: Introduction   1

Chapter 1   Bicycle and helmet use of adolescents:
We need to study it again   3
Ronald Chow and Joav Merrick

Chapter 2   Bicycle and helmet use:
The survey instrument   7
Ronald Chow

Section two: Ontario   13

Chapter 3   Helmet use of adolescents at Ashbury
College in Ottawa, Canada   15
*Ronald Chow, Michael Borean,
Drew Hollenberg, Jaclyn Viehweger,
Kendal Young, Andrew Young,
Brian Storosko and Norman Southward*

Contents

Chapter 4	Helmet use of adolescents at Linden School in Toronto, Canada *Ronald Chow, Michael Borean,* *Drew Hollenberg, Jaclyn Viehweger,* *Beth Alexander and Janice Gladstone*	**23**
Chapter 5	Helmet use of adolescents at Crestwood Preparatory College in Toronto, Canada *Ronald Chow, Michael Borean,* *Drew Hollenberg, Jaclyn Viehweger,* *and Dave Hecock*	**31**
Chapter 6	Helmet use of adolescents at Elmwood School in Ottawa, Canada *Ronald Chow, Michael Borean,* *Drew Hollenberg, Jaclyn Viehweger,* *James Whitehouse and Cheryl Boughton*	**41**
Section three: British Columbia		**51**
Chapter 7	Helmet use of adolescents at Aberdeen Hall in Kelowna, Canada *Ronald Chow, Michael Borean,* *Drew Hollenberg, Jaclyn Viehweger* *and Jerry Hesse*	**53**
Chapter 8	Helmet use of adolescents at Southridge School in Surrey, Canada *Ronald Chow, Michael Borean,* *Drew Hollenberg and Jaclyn Viehweger*	**61**
Chapter 9	Helmet use of adolescents in the Province of British Columbia, Canada *Jaclyn Viehweger, Michael Borean,* *Drew Hollenberg, Sandro Cuzzetto* *and Ronald Chow*	**71**

Contents

Section four: United States of America		**79**
Chapter 10	Helmet use of adolescents at Avon Old Farms School in Avon, United States *Ronald Chow, Jaclyn Viehweger, Michael Borean and Drew Hollenberg*	**81**
Section five: Overall		**91**
Chapter 11	Bicycle and helmet use of adolescents: A meta-analysis *Ronald Chow, Michael Borean, Drew Hollenberg, Jaclyn Viehweger, Tharani Anpalagan and Anna Rzepka*	**93**
Section six: Acknowledgments		**109**
Chapter 12	About the editors	**111**
Chapter 13	About Infinitas Research Group, London, Ontario, Canada	**115**
Chapter 14	About the Bicycle Safety and Awareness Club, London, Ontario, Canada	**117**
Chapter 15	About the National Institute of Child Health and Human Development in Israel	**119**
Chapter 16	About the book series "Pediatrics, child and adolescent health"	**125**
Section seven: Index		**131**
Index		**133**

Section one: Introduction

In: Bicycles
Editors: Ronald Chow et al.

ISBN: 978-1-53612-458-3
© 2017 Nova Science Publishers, Inc.

Chapter 1

BICYCLE AND HELMET USE OF ADOLESCENTS: WE NEED TO STUDY IT AGAIN

Ronald Chow[1,], BMSc(C) and Joav Merrick[2-6], MD, MMedSc, DMSc*

[1]Infinitas Research Group, London, Ontario, Canada
[2]National Institute of Child Health and Human Development, Jerusalem, Israel
[3]Office of the Medical Director, Health Services, Division for Intellectual and Developmental Disabilities, Ministry of Social Affairs and Social Services, Jerusalem, Israel
[4]Division of Pediatrics, Hadassah Hebrew University Medical Centre, Mt Scopus Campus, Jerusalem, Israel

---

* Correspondence: Ronald Chow BMSc(C), Bicycle Safety and Awareness Club, London, Ontario, Canada. Email: rchow48@uwo.ca.

[5]Kentucky Children's Hospital, University of Kentucky College of
Medicine, Lexington, Kentucky, United States
[6]Center for Healthy Development, School of Public Health,
Georgia State University, Atlanta, United States

> Helmet use can substantially reduce the risks associated with bicycle injuries, as these protective devices can prevent an array of serious facial injuries. A meta-analysis was carried out looking to summarize studies into the helmet use of adolescents and young adults, where we found a U-trend between age and helmet use, with proportion of individuals regularly wearing a helmet declining first and then rising with reference to progression of age. The increasing trend in young adults has been well-documented in the literature, but few studies have looked into the helmet use among adolescents. In this book produced in collaboration with the Bicycle Safety and Awareness Club in Ontario, Canada, we present survey studies conducted in independent schools in North America, looking into bicycle and helmet use of adolescents.

INTRODUCTION

A meta-analysis was carried out looking to summarize studies into the helmet use of adolescents and young adults (1). A U-trend was noted between age and helmet use, with proportion of individuals regularly wearing a helmet declining first and then rising with reference to progression of age. The increasing trend in young adults has been well-documented in the literature, with 13 papers looking into the topic and verifying the trend (2-14). However, only four studies have looked into the helmet use among adolescents (15-18).

A survey circulated to Grade 7 to 12 students and inquiring about helmet use of adolescent cyclists at an all-boys independent day school in Toronto, Canada was published (15), and reported a negative correlation. Among school cyclists, 96%, 76% and 59% of students in Grade 7 and 8, Grade 9 and 10, and Grade 11 and 12, respectively, used helmets regularly. For recreational cyclists, 88%, 60% and 58% of the same groups used a helmet frequently (15).

Borean et al. (16) also recorded a correlation amongst high school students in Markham, Canada in their survey study. Helmet-use rates for public high school students were 14% and 30% amongst cyclists who commute to school, and 41% and 38% for those who used their bicycle during their recreational time (16). Studies by Anpalagan et al. (17) and Borean et al. (18) also verified the trend in a public co-educational school and an independent co-educational school.

Even though the trend was verified, there exists notable variation between different sample populations. Given that some of the previous findings noted a borderline trend, there may exist the possibility that variations noted in other geographical regions may lead to a lack of detection of a negative correlation. There therefore needs to be further studies looking into helmet use of the adolescent population to further look into the proposed negative correlation trend.

REFERENCES

[1] Chow R. Bicycle and helmet use of young adults and adolescents: a meta-analysis. Int J Child Health Hum Dev 2018;11(1), in press.

[2] Chow R, Borean M, Hollenberg D, Ganguli N, Freedman Z, Kang R, et al. Helmet use of young adults in New York State, United States of America. Int J Child Health Hum Dev 2018;11(1), in press.

[3] Anpalagan T, Hollenberg D, Borean M, Rzepka A, Chow R. Helmet use of young adults in London, Canada. Int J Child Health Hum Dev 2018;11(1), in press.

[4] Anpalagan T, Panigrahi I, Borean M, Hollenberg D, Rzepka A, Viehweger J et al. Helmet use of young adults in Hamilton, Canada. Int J Child Health Hum Dev 2018;11(1); in press.

[5] Rzepka A, Borean M, Hollenberg D, Chan Z, Binns A, Weise E, et al. Helmet use of young adults in Guelph, Canada. Int J Child Health Hum Dev 2018;11(1); in press.

[6] Anpalagan T, Duarte N, Borean M, Anpalagan J, Camilleri R, Hollenberg D, et al. Helmet use of young adults in Waterloo, Canada. Int J Child Health Hum Dev 2018;11(1), in press.

[7] Chow R, Borean M, Hollenberg D, Ho C, Ng W, Guo W, et al. Helmet use of young adults in Toronto, Canada. Int J Child Health Hum Dev 2018;11(1), in press.
[8] Viehweger J, Borean M, Tang M, Hollenberg D, Anpalagan T, Rzepka A, et al. Helmet use of young adults in St. Catherines, Canada. Int J Child Health Hum Dev 2018;11(1), in press.
[9] Viehweger J, Borean M, Midroni L, Midroni C, Hollenberg D, Anpalagan T et al. Helmet use of young adults in Kingston, Canada. Int J Child Health Hum Dev 2018;11(1), in press.
[10] Chow R, Borean M, Hollenberg D, Song K, Liu J, Young T, et al. Helmet use of young adults in Montreal, Canada. Int J Child Health Hum Dev 2018;11(1), in press.
[11] Chow R, Rzepka A, Borean M, Parekh R, Hollenberg D, Anpalagan T, et al. Helmet use of young adults in Saskatoon, Canada. Int J Child Health Hum Dev 2018;11(1), in press.
[12] Hollenberg D, Ferguson T, Borean M, Anpalagan T, Rzepka A, Viehweger J, et al. Helmet use of young adults in Halifax, Canada. Int J Child Health Hum Dev 2018;11(1), in press.
[13] Chow R, Borean M, Murai A, Menon G, Hollenberg D, Anpalagan T, et al. Helmet use of young adults in California, United States of America. Int J Child Health Hum Dev 2018;11(1): in press.
[14] Chow R, Hollenberg D, Borean M, Goh S, Anpalagan T, Rzepka A, et al. Helmet use of young adults in Dublin, Ireland. Int J Child Health Hum Dev 2018;11(1), in press.
[15] Chow R, Hollenberg D, Pintilie A, Midroni C, Cumner S. Helmet use of adolescent cyclists at Crescent School in Toronto, Canada. Int J Adolesc Med Health 2016; in press.
[16] Borean M, Ho S, Hollenberg D, Anpalagan T, Rzepka A, Viehweger J, et al. Helmet use of adolescents in Markham, Canada. Int J Adolesc Med Health 2017; in press.
[17] Anpalagan T, Borean M, Chen L, Viehweger J, Hollenberg D, Rzepka A, et al. Helmet use of adolescents in Toronto, Canada. Int J Child Health Hum Dev 2018;11(1), in press.
[18] Borean M, Trasente V, Rzepka A, Viggiani D, Viotto D, Hollenberg D, et al. Helmet use of adolescents at De La Salle Oaklands in Toronto, Canada. Int J Child Health Hum Dev 2018;11(1), in press.

In: Bicycles
Editors: Ronald Chow et al.

ISBN: 978-1-53612-458-3
© 2017 Nova Science Publishers, Inc.

Chapter 2

BICYCLE AND HELMET USE: THE SURVEY INSTRUMENT

Ronald Chow, BMSc(C)*
Bicycle Safety and Awareness Club, London, Ontario, Canada

The Bicycle Safety and Awareness Club has previously looked into bicycle safety practices of adolescents and young adults across the world. A standardized questionnaire was used to survey the safety practices of adolescents at independent schools.

INTRODUCTION

The Bicycle Safety and Awareness Club has previously looked into bicycle safety practices of adolescents and young adults across the

---

* Correspondence: Ronald Chow BMSc(C), Bicycle Safety and Awareness Club, London, Ontario, Canada. Email: rchow48@uwo.ca.

world. In this collection, a standardized questionnaire was used to survey the safety practices of adolescents at independent schools.

THE SURVEY

The questionnaire for adolescents queried about school-grade. The second question on the first page was a Yes/No question regarding whether the participant commutes to school using a bicycle; should they answer “Yes”, they would have been re-directed to page 2, while an answer of “No” directs them to progress to page 3 (see Figure 1). The second page of the questionnaire for adolescents asked participants about the duration of a typical ride to school, the frequency at which they commute, frequency for which they use a helmet, and whether they are aware of the legislation in Ontario regarding mandatory helmet use; there is also a short-answer question asking for reasons why individuals choose not to wear helmets (see Figure 2).

Bicycle and Helmet Use

Please note that this form is anonymous.

* Required

What grade are you in? *

Grade 7
Grade 8
Grade 9
Grade 10
Grade 11
Grade 12

Have you ever used a bike to commute to school? *

Yes
No

Continue »

25% completed

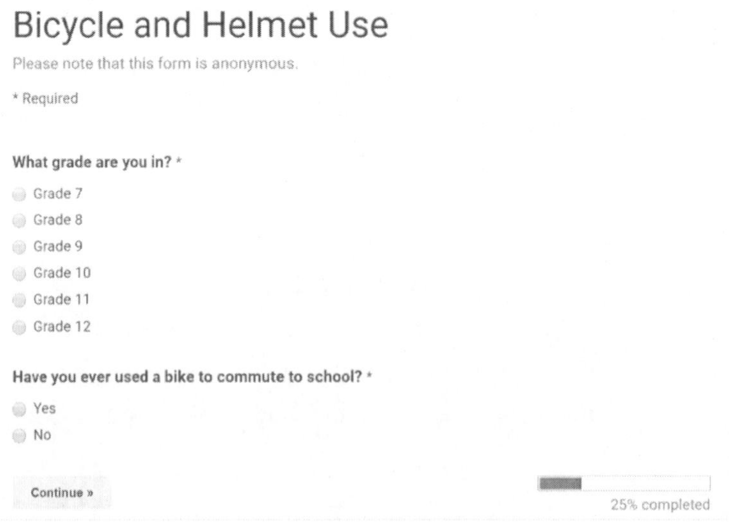

Figure 1. Survey (page 1).

Bicycle and helmet use 9

The third page has another Yes/No question asking whether an adolescent uses a bike during their recreational time; as with the prior Yes/No question, an answer of "Yes" progressed the participant to page 4 whereas an answer of "No" brought the survey to an end (see Figure 3). The fourth page investigated into the frequency of helmet use during recreational cycling, reasons for not using a helmet, and inquired about the knowledge of bicycle legislation (see Figure 4).

Bicycle and Helmet Use
* Required

Bicycle and Helmet Use On The Commute To School

How long is the bike ride? *
- Under 10 minutes
- 10-20 minutes
- 20-30 minutes
- Over 30 minutes

How often do you commute to school via bike? *
- Always (100%)
- Often (75%-99%)
- Sometimes (50%-74%)
- On Occasion (25%-49%)
- Rarely (0%-24%)

When you bike, how often do you wear a helmet? *
- Always (100%)
- Often (75%-99%)
- Sometimes (50%-74%)
- On Occasion (25%-49%)
- Rarely (0%-24%)

Why do you not wear a helmet?
Only applicable for those who do not answer "Always"

True or False: It is required by law that you wear a helmet. *
- True
- False

« Back   Continue »

50% completed

Figure 2. Survey (page 2).

Bicycle and Helmet Use
* Required

Please note that this form is anonymous.

Do you use your bike in your recreational time (outside of school)? *
- Yes
- No

[« Back] [Continue »]   75% completed

Figure 3. Survey (page 3).

Bicycle and Helmet Use
* Required

Bicycle and Helmet Use During Recreational Time

When you bike, how often do you wear a helmet? *
- Always (100%)
- Often (75%-99%)
- Sometimes (50%-74%)
- On Occasion (25%-49%)
- Rarely (0%-24%)

Why do you not wear a helmet?
Only applicable for those who do not answer "Always"

[text box]

True or False: It is required by law that you wear a helmet. *
- True
- False

[« Back] [Submit]   100%: You made it.
Never submit passwords through Google Forms.

Figure 4. Survey (page 4).

For the statistical analyses of the collected data, responses for questions on page 2 and 4 of both questionnaires were collapsed into a few categories. For the question about duration of bicycle commute to school/university, the responses were grouped into "Under 20 Minutes" and "Over 20 Minutes." The questions regarding frequency (of commute, and of helmet use) were similarly grouped into two responses "Always/Often" and "Rarely/On Occasion/Sometimes." The resulting contingency tables for the multiple-choice questions were analyzed using the Statistical Analysis Software (Version 9.4 for Windows), via the Fisher exact test. The reason(s) provided by recreational and student cyclists for lack of helmet use was conveyed via descriptive statistics.

Section Two: Ontario

In: Bicycles
Editors: Ronald Chow et al.
ISBN: 978-1-53612-458-3
© 2017 Nova Science Publishers, Inc.

Chapter 3

HELMET USE OF ADOLESCENTS AT ASHBURY COLLEGE IN OTTAWA, CANADA

Ronald Chow[1,], BMSc(C), Michael Borean[1], BMSc(C), Drew Hollenberg[1], BMSc(C), Jaclyn Viehweger[1], BMSc(C), Kendal Young[2], MA, Andrew Young[2], MEd, Brian Storosko[2], MEd and Norman Southward[2], MEd*

[1]Bicycle Safety and Awareness Club, London, Ontario, Canada
[2]Ashbury College, Ottawa, Ontario, Canada

There are currently four published studies looking into helmet use of adolescents. However, these are all based in Toronto, Canada. A prior meta-analysis has noted that there is variation by geographical region among the young adult population, and hence adolescents in other regions may similarly use helmets at a different frequency. The aim of this study was to look into helmet use of adolescents in Ottawa, Canada. A

---

[*] Correspondence: Ronald Chow BMSc(C), Bicycle Safety and Awareness Club, London, Ontario, Canada. Email: rchow48@uwo.ca.

questionnaire was circulated to Grade 7 and 8 students at Ashbury College, an independent co-educational day school in Ottawa, Canada. The primary objectives of the survey were to determine (1) the percentage of cyclists at the school and (2) the percentage of cyclists who wear a helmet. The proportion of individuals who frequently use a helmet and proportion of individuals who are aware are approximately equal. However, this is a correlation and not necessarily a causation. The helmet use rate for school commuters, 76%, is slightly lower than the rates noted in prior studies. It is comforting to note that the majority of student cyclists do not regularly commute to school, so the low helmet-use rate may simply be a phenomenon of lack of regular commute. Educational and encouragement programs could still be employed to hopefully raise this lower rate.

INTRODUCTION

A study was completed at Crescent School, an independent school in Toronto, Canada, looking into bicycle safety practices of adolescent boys. The authors surveyed Grade 7 to 12 students and reported a negative correlation between helmet use and age. While students aged 13 and 14 years old used a helmet 96% of the time, those in the 15-16 years old and 17-18 years old cohort only used a helmet 76% and 59%, respectively (1).

Many follow-up studies were conducted in the young adult population to look into whether this trend persists in the young adult population. According to a recent meta-analysis, there currently exists thirteen studies looking into this topic in the young adult population. The quality and quantity of past studies have resulted in the detection of a general trend among young adults that helmet-usage is at an all-time low among 18 to 19 years old, but increases as young adults mature (2). The meta-analysis also revealed that only the trend initially uncovered by Chow et al. (1) seems to prevail among adolescents. However, there were only four published studies looking into helmet use of adolescents (1, 3-5).

The four studies in the literature looked into the safety practices of adolescents in Toronto, Canada, but only four studies have looked into and concurred with the initial trend. The prior meta-analysis has noted that there is variation by geographical region (2), and hence adolescents in other regions may use helmets at a different frequency. The aim of this study was to look into helmet use of adolescents in Ottawa, Canada.

OUR STUDY

A questionnaire was circulated to Grade 7 and 8 students at Ashbury College, an independent co-educational day school in Ottawa, Canada. The primary objectives of the survey were to determine 1) the percentage of cyclists at the school and 2) the percentage of cyclists who wear a helmet. The questionnaire posed questions regarding bicycle-use in two main instances - the first instance was centred around bicycle-use as a means of transportation to arrive at the school, and the second focused on bicycle-use during recreational time. The secondary objective of the questionnaire was to determine the reasoning or motive of those who do not wear helmets, and subsequently gauge the students' knowledge on legislation around helmet-use. The questionnaire was anonymous, and students were strongly encouraged to complete the survey (6).

The results of the questionnaire were examined by cohorts of grades - Grade 7 and Grade 8. For questions pertaining to frequency of commute and frequency of helmet use, results were collapsed to yield two responses - "Always/Often" and "Rarely/On Occasion/Sometimes." The duration of the commute to school was also divided into two responses - "Under 20 minutes" and "Over 20 minutes." Fisher-exact test was used to examine the difference in proportions for multiple-choice results. Descriptive statistics were used for the short-answer question inquiring about helmet use. All analyses were performed using the Statistical Analysis Software (SAS Version 9.4 for Windows) (6).

FINDINGS

A total of 82 students completed the survey, of which 41 identified as Grade 7 students and 41 reported that they were in Grade 8. 34% of Grade 7s and 38% of Grade 8s remarked that they have cycled to school (p=0.6416). The majority of students - all of Grade 7 students and 80% of Grade 8 students - have commute times of under 20 minutes via bike (p=0.2241). The vast majority of students do not regularly commute to school (p=0.3295; 79% for Grade 7s and 93% for Grade 8s). Grade 7 and 8 students wear helmets at approximately equivalent rates (p=0.9999), at 79% and 73%, respectively. In corollary, their awareness of a legislation that mandates helmet use is about the same - 87% of Grade 8 and 71% of Grade 7 students noted that there is a law (p=0.3898) (see Table 1).

Table 1. Demographics of cyclists to school

	Grade 7	Grade 8	*p*-value
Cyclist/Non-Cyclist			0.6416
Cyclist	14 (34%)	15 (37%)	
Non-Cyclist	27 (66%)	26 (63%)	
Duration			0.2241
Under 20 min	14 (100%)	12 (80%)	
Over 20 min	0 (0%)	3 (20%)	
Frequency of commute			0.3295
Always/Often	3 (21%)	1 (7%)	
Rarely/On Occasion/Sometimes	11 (79%)	14 (93%)	
Frequency of helmet use			0.9999
Always/Often	11 (79%)	11 (73%)	
Rarely/On Occasion/Sometimes	3 (21%)	4 (27%)	
Legislation about helmet use			0.3898
True	10 (71%)	13 (87%)	
False	4 (29%)	2 (13%)	

A high proportion of Grade 7 (83%) and Grade 8 (90%) students regarded themselves as recreational cyclists (p=0.5187). The majority of recreational cyclists, regardless of age, utilized a helmet often (p=0.7617); 79% of Grade 7 and 84% of Grade 8 students use a helmet when cycling recreationally. The two age cohorts were aware of the legislation at a 76% and 89% rate (p=0.2090) (see Table 2).

Table 2. Demographics of recreational cyclists

	Grade 7	Grade 8	*p*-value
Cyclist/Non-Cyclist			0.5187
Cyclist	34 (83%)	37 (90%)	
Non-Cyclist	7 (17%)	4 (10%)	
Frequency of helmet use			0.7617
Always/Often	27 (79%)	31 (84%)	
Rarely/On Occasion/Sometimes	7 (21%)	6 (16%)	
Legislation about helmet use			0.2090
True	26 (76%)	33 (89%)	
False	8 (24%)	4 (11%)	

Table 3. Reasons for not wearing a helmet - school commute

Reasons	Grade 7	Grade 8
Short and safe commute	1 (33%)	1 (14%)
I'm a confident biker	1 (33%)	1 (14%)
I forget	1 (33%)	2 (29%)
I'm worried about losing it	0 (0%)	1 (14%)
Helmet is too small	0 (0%)	2 (29%)

Three Grade 7 students who cycle to school provided a reason for not using a helmet. One noted that they have a short and safe commute, another one regarded themselves as a good biker, and the third noted that they forget to use a helmet. The most common reasons provided by Grade 8 students are that their helmet is too small (29%) and that they forget (29%); other reasons included that it is a short commute (14%), they are a safe/confident cyclist (14%), and that they worry about losing their helmet after the commute (14%) (see Table 3).

For recreational cycling, 11 reasons were provided by Grade 7 students and 12 explanations were offered by Grade 8 students as to why they do not wear a helmet. The most common reason provided by the younger age group was that they are a safe cyclist and hence do not need a helmet (36%). Successively popular reasons were that they do not know where their helmet is (18%), it is uncomfortable or does not look aesthetically pleasing (18%), they ride a very short distance or do not ride often (18%), and that they simply forget (9%). The 12 responses provided by Grade 8 students were distributed equally across six explanations (17% each) - they are a safe cyclist, they do not know where their helmet is, a helmet does not look good, they forget to wear one, it is a short ride, and other (i.e., they are afraid someone will steal it) (see Table 4).

Table 4. Reasons for not wearing a helmet - recreational cycling

Reasons	Grade 7	Grade 8
I'm a safe cyclist	4 (36%)	2 (17%)
I don't know where it is	2 (18%)	2 (17%)
Doesn't look good/ uncomfortable	2 (18%)	2 (17%)
I forget to wear one	1 (9%)	2 (17%)
It's a short ride/ don't ride often	2 (18%)	2 (17%)
Other*	0 (0%)	2 (17%)

*Other: "I don't need one," "Afraid someone will steal it."

DISCUSSION

The results are rather encouraging with respect to frequency of helmet use and knowledge of legislation - the frequency and awareness level are approximately equivalent within age cohorts. This finding suggests that all those students who know there exists a law use a helmet. However, such a finding should be carefully interpreted as this is a correlation and not a causation.

The conglomerate helmet use rate for school-commuters (22/29, or 76%) is slightly lower than the rates noted in two prior studies (96% reported by Chow et al. (1) and 80% recorded by Borean et al. (5)) of a similar age cohort at other independent schools. Educational and encouragement programs could be employed to hopefully raise this lower rate. However, it is comforting to note that the majority of student cyclists do not regularly commute to school, so the low helmet-use rate may simply be a phenomenon of lack of regular commute.

The helmet-use rate of recreational cyclists (58/71, or 82%) is on-par with the previous two studies. The study conducted among adolescent boys noted a 88% rate (1), while another study carried out among adolescent boys and girls at a co-educational institution informed about a 74% rate (5). The meta-analysis conducted by Chow also revealed that the rate among adolescent girls was 84% (2). Students at Ashbury College hence have similar helmet-wearing rates as other independent schools. These rates, as are all other rates revealed in prior studies, are far from perfect, which further supports the suggestion for the implementation of more educational and encouragement programs surrounding the benefits of helmet use.

This study was not without limitations. As with any survey, there exists the possibility of a response bias. Additionally, as the survey was circulated around to students via media networks and advertised as optional, there also exists the potential for a sampling bias. These biases were hopefully minimized by accruing a substantial sample size, but p-values yielded should still be interpreted with caution.

In conclusion, the proportion of individuals who frequently use a helmet and the proportion of individuals who are aware are approximately equal. However, this is a correlation and not necessarily a causation. The helmet use rate for school commuters, 76%, is slightly lower than the rates noted in prior studies. It is comforting to note that the majority of student cyclists do not regularly commute to school, so the low helmet-use rate may simply be a phenomenon of lack of regular commute. Educational and encouragement programs could still be employed to hopefully raise this lower rate.

Acknowledgments

We would like to thank all of those who participated in the questionnaire.

References

[1] Chow R, Hollenberg D, Pintilie A, Midroni C, Cumner S. Helmet use of adolescent cyclists at Crescent School in Toronto, Canada. Int J Adolesc Med Health 2016; in press.
[2] Chow R. Bicycle and helmet use of young adults and adolescents: a meta-analysis. Int J Child Health Hum Dev 2018;11(1), in press.
[3] Borean M, Ho S, Hollenberg D, Anpalagan T, Rzepka A, Viehweger J, et al. Helmet use of adolescents in Markham, Canada. Int J Adolesc Med Health 2017, in press.
[4] Anpalagan T, Borean M, Chen L, Viehweger J, Hollenberg D, Rzepka A, et al. Helmet use of adolescents in Toronto, Canada. Int J Child Health Hum Dev 2018;11(1), in press.
[5] Borean M, Trasente V, Rzepka A, Viggiani D, Viotto D, Hollenberg D, et al. Helmet use of adolescents at De La Salle Oaklands in Toronto, Canada. Int J Child Health Hum Dev 2018;11(1), in press.
[6] Chow R. Bicycle and helmet use: the survey instrument. Int J Child Health Hum Dev 2019; in press.

In: Bicycles
Editors: Ronald Chow et al.
ISBN: 978-1-53612-458-3
© 2017 Nova Science Publishers, Inc.

Chapter 4

HELMET USE OF ADOLESCENTS AT LINDEN SCHOOL IN TORONTO, CANADA

Ronald Chow[1,], BMSc(C),*
Michael Borean[1], BMSc(C),
Drew Hollenberg[1], BMSc(C),
Jaclyn Viehweger[1], BMSc(C),
Beth Alexander[2], MA
and Janice Gladstone[2], MASc

[1]Bicycle Safety and Awareness Club, London, Ontario, Canada
[2]Linden School, Toronto, Ontario, Canada

A study revealed a negative correlation between age and helmet use - as students matured, helmet use fell from 96% to 59%. While the negative correlation has been studied on five occasions in a co-ed school, it was only studied once in a single-sex school environment - in the original

---

[*] Correspondence: Ronald Chow BMSc(C), Bicycle Safety and Awareness Club, London, Ontario, Canada. Email: rchow48@uwo.ca.

study at Crescent School. It has never been studied at an all-girls school; there may exist some difference in rates, similar to how there is variation between Crescent School and the other schools. The aim of this study was to determine the helmet-use rates of adolescent girls at Linden School in Toronto, Canada. A questionnaire was circulated to Grade 7-12 students at Linden School in Toronto, Canada. The results suggest that there does exist a negative correlation with respect to age and helmet use. Even with the small sample size and corresponding limited statistical power, the negative correlation noted in an all-boys population and co-educational environment has also been observed in the all-girls adolescent population. Future studies should look into repeating such a sample among a larger all-girl population to confirm the observations contained within.

INTRODUCTION

Six studies (1-6) have examined the biking practices of high school students. The original study conducted at an all-boys school in Toronto noted a negative correlation between age and helmet use (1) - as students matured, helmet use fell from 96% to 59%. Other studies conducted at co-educational schools failed to disprove the trend (2-6), with many in fact confirming the observation.

The overall picture, as provided by Chow in a meta-analysis (7), suggests that the observation noted in the original study may permeate among the adolescent population. However, the review also showed that there does exist variation in helmet-use rates as reported by different studies.

While the negative correlation has been studied on five occasions in a co-ed school, it was only studied once in a single-sex school environment - in the original study at Crescent School. It has never been studied at an all-girls school; there may exist some difference in rates, similar to how there is variation between Crescent School and the other schools. The aim of this study was to determine the helmet-use rates of adolescent girls at Linden School in Toronto, Canada.

OUR STUDY

The questionnaire was circulated to Grade 7 through 12 students at Linden School, an independent all-girls day school in Toronto, Canada. The primary objectives of the survey were to determine (1) the percentage of cyclists at the school and (2) among those cyclists, the percentage who frequently wear a helmet. The questionnaire posed questions regarding bicycle-use on two occasions - the first instance was centred around bicycle-use as a means of transportation to arrive at the school, and the second focused on bicycle-use during recreational time. The secondary objective of the questionnaire was to determine the reasoning or motive of those who do not wear helmets, and subsequently gauge the students' knowledge on legislation around helmet-use. The questionnaire was anonymous, and students were strongly encouraged to complete the survey (8).

The data was analyzed by age - Grade 7 and 8, Grade 9 and 10, Grade 11 and 12. For questions pertaining to frequency of commute and frequency of helmet use, results were collapsed to yield two responses - "Always/Often" and "Rarely/On Occasion/Sometimes." The duration of the commute to school was also divided into two responses - "Under 20 minutes" and "Over 20 minutes." Fisher-exact test was used to examine the difference in proportions for multiple-choice results. Descriptive statistics were used for the short-answer question inquiring about helmet use. All analyses were performed using the Statistical Analysis Software (SAS Version 9.4 for Windows) (8).

FINDINGS

26 adolescents filled out the questionnaire. 10 identified as Grade 7 and 8 students, 7 as Grade 9 and 10, and 9 as Grade 11 and 12 students. Only a few students identified themselves as individuals who have

cycled to school - 20% of Grade 7 and 8, 14% of Grade 9 and 10, and 33% of Grade 11 and 12 students (p=0.7209). Most of the commute lengths were over 20 minutes (p=0.9999), and all of these students do not regularly commute via bike (p=0.9999). It seems that the older students do not use a helmet as often (33% compared to 100%), and that they are less aware that there exists a legislation mandating helmet use for adolescents (33% compared to 100%) (see Table 1).

Table 1. Demographics of cyclists to school

	Grades 7 & 8	Grades 9 & 10	Grades 11 & 12	*p*-value
Cyclist/Non-Cyclist				0.7209
Cyclist	2 (20%)	1 (14%)	3 (33%)	
Non-Cyclist	8 (80%)	6 (86%)	6 (67%)	
Duration				0.9999
Under 20 min	0 (0%)	0 (0%)	1 (33%)	
Over 20 min	2 (100%)	1 (100%)	2 (67%)	
Frequency of commute				0.9999
Always/Often	0 (0%)	0 (0%)	0 (0%)	
Rarely/On Occasion/Sometimes	2 (100%)	1 (100%)	3 (100%)	
Frequency of helmet use				0.5999
Always/Often	2 (100%)	1 (100%)	1 (33%)	
Rarely/On Occasion/Sometimes	0 (0%)	0 (0%)	2 (67%)	
Legislation about helmet use				0.5999
True	2 (100%)	1 (100%)	1 (33%)	
False	0 (0%)	0 (0%)	2 (67%)	

There seems to exist a trend that a smaller proportion of older students who noted that they use their bike during their recreational time (p=0.2133). There exists a negative correlation between helmet use and age (p=0.0165); while 100% of Grade 7 and 8 students regularly used a helmet, only 83% and 40% of Grade 9 and 10 and Grade 11 and

12 students, respectively. The data also reveals that the older cohort is less knowledgeable about the legislation requiring adolescents to wear helmets when riding their bike (p=0.0273), with only 20% compared to 89% of students acknowledging a legislation exists (see Table 2).

Table 2. Demographics of recreational cyclists

	Grades 7 & 8	Grades 9 & 10	Grades 11 & 12	*p*-value
Cyclist/Non-Cyclist				0.2133
Cyclist	9 (90%)	6 (86%)	5 (56%)	
Non-Cyclist	1 (10%)	1 (14%)	4 (44%)	
Frequency of helmet use				0.0165
Always/Often	9 (100%)	5 (83%)	2 (40%)	
Rarely/On Occasion/Sometimes	0 (0%)	1 (17%)	3 (60%)	
Legislation about helmet use				0.0273
True	8 (89%)	5 (83%)	1 (20%)	
False	1 (11%)	1 (17%)	4 (80%)	

The two students who did not regularly use a helmet when commuting to school did not provide a reason for not using a helmet. Among the sample population of recreational cyclists, six reasons were provided in total, two from each age cohort. Half of the Grade 7 and 8, and Grade 11 and 12 group, and all of the Grade 9 and 10 students, noted that they do not use a helmet because they ride on a safe/short path. Other reasons included the mention that their helmet was broken (50% of Grade 7 and 8), and that they do not own one (50% of Grade 11 and 12) (see Table 3).

Table 3. Reasons for not wearing a helmet - recreational cycling

Reasons	Grades 7 & 8	Grades 9 & 10	Grades 11 & 12
Broken	1 (50%)	0 (0%)	0 (0%)
Safe/short biking path	1 (50%)	2 (100%)	1 (50%)
Do not own one	0 (0%)	0 (0%)	1 (50%)

DISCUSSION

The sample size of this study was the smallest compared to the six prior studies looking into helmet use of adolescents. This is a result of a small school population. Nevertheless, the study was still able to confirm prior observations that there exists a negative correlation with respect to age and helmet use.

There also seems to be a lack of awareness of the law with respect to helmet use among the older cohort. This may hence explain why the older cohort does not use a helmet as frequently, as they do not believe there exists a law mandating it. Educational programs could be designed to increase the awareness of this legislation and hopefully increase the use of helmets.

Educational programs could also be directed to informing adolescents that although they may be strong cyclists, the possibility of a collision and head injury is always present. A mechanical failure with the bike, or even a human error by surrounding individuals, could quickly result in an accident in which a helmet could hopefully reduce the trauma experienced by the subject. These two aspects of education, legislation and possibility of injury, would hopefully increase the proportion of individuals who regularly use a helmet.

This study was not without limitations. The sample size was small and hence did not lead to high statistical power. However, the results still allowed for the detection of the negative correlation trend. Also, as a result of the nature of the survey methods, there exists the possibility of both a response and sampling bias.

In conclusion, this study suggests that there does exist a negative correlation with respect to age and helmet use. Even with the small sample size and corresponding limited statistical power, the negative correlation noted in an all-boys population and co-educational environment has also been observed in the all-girls adolescent population. Future studies should look into repeating such a sample among a larger sample size of all-girls population to confirm the observations contained within.

ACKNOWLEDGMENTS

We would like to thank all of those who participated in the questionnaire.

REFERENCES

[1] Chow R, Hollenberg D, Pintilie A, Midroni C, Cumner S. Helmet use of adolescent cyclists at Crescent School in Toronto, Canada. Int J Adolesc Med Health 2016, in press.
[2] Borean M, Ho S, Hollenberg D, Anpalagan T, Rzepka A, Viehweger J, et al. Helmet use of adolescents in Markham, Canada. Int J Adolesc Med Health 2017, in press.
[3] Anpalagan T, Borean M, Chen L, Viehweger J, Hollenberg D, Rzepka A, et al. Helmet use of adolescents in Toronto, Canada. Int J Child Health Hum Dev 2018;11(1), in press.
[4] Borean M, Trasente V, Rzepka A, Viggiani D, Viotto D, Hollenberg D, et al. Helmet use of adolescents at De La Salle Oaklands in Toronto, Canada. Int J Child Health Hum Dev 2018;11(1), in press.
[5] Chow R, Borean M, Hollenberg D, Viehweger J, Young K, Southward N. Helmet use of adolescents at Ashbury College in Ottawa, Canada. Int J Child Health Hum Dev 2019, in press.
[6] Chow R, Borean M, Hollenberg D, Viehweger J, Hesse J. Helmet use of adolescents at Aberdeen Hall in Kelowna, Canada. Int J Child Health Hum Dev 2019, in press.
[7] Chow R. Bicycle and helmet use of young adults and adolescents: A meta-analysis. Int J Child Health Hum Dev 2018;11(1), in press.
[8] Chow R. Bicycle and helmet use: the survey instrument. Int J Child Health Hum Dev 2019, in press.

In: Bicycles
Editors: Ronald Chow et al.

ISBN: 978-1-53612-458-3
© 2017 Nova Science Publishers, Inc.

Chapter 5

HELMET USE OF ADOLESCENTS AT CRESTWOOD PREPARATORY COLLEGE IN TORONTO, CANADA

Ronald Chow[1,]*, BMSc(C),
Michael Borean[1], BMSc(C),
Drew Hollenberg[1], BMSc(C),
Jaclyn Viehweger[1], BMSc(C)
and Dave Hecock[2], MEd

[1]Bicycle Safety and Awareness Club, London, Ontario, Canada
[2]Crestwood Preparatory School, Toronto, Ontario, Canada

The aim of this chapter was to look into the rate of helmet use at a co-educational independent school in Toronto, Canada. The standardized questionnaire (25) was circulated to Grade 7 through 12 students at Crestwood Preparatory College, an independent co-educational day

---

* Correspondence: Ronald Chow BMSc(C), Bicycle Safety and Awareness Club, London, Ontario, Canada. Email: rchow48@uwo.ca.

school in Toronto, Canada. The primary objectives of the survey were to determine 1) the percentage of cyclists at the school and 2) among those cyclists, the percentage who frequently wear a helmet. A total of 77 responses were collected, of which 26 noted that they were in Grade 7-8, 32 in Grade 9-10 and 19 in Grade 11-12. This study failed to record a negative correlation between age and bicycle helmet use. This may be a result of different upbringings of adolescents in this population. Additionally, the percentage of individuals who are aware of the legislation is lower than the proportion of those who regularly wear a helmet. In order to improve the frequency of helmet use, educational programs could be employed to increase the awareness of the legislation of helmet use. This could lead to more students being aware of the implications of not wearing a helmet should law enforcement investigate into them, and resultantly a higher percentage of students wearing a helmet. The programs could also further emphasize the efficacy of helmets.

INTRODUCTION

Helmet use has been well-documented among the young adult population (1-13), with a meta-analysis of all published studies (14) suggesting that there exists a positive correlation with age among the young adult population - as young adults mature, the proportion of people who regularly use a helmet increases. While it was well-documented amongst that population, only four studies looking into helmet use of adolescents were included in the meta-analysis (15-18).

The general trend in adolescents is different than that in young adults; in adolescents, there seems to exist a negative correlation. Many studies, in addition to the four in the meta-analysis (19-24), have looked into the helmet use rates and noted that as adolescents age, helmet use decreases. While the trend seems to hold regardless of geographic location, there seems to exist variation across the studies. The aim of this study was to look into the rate of helmet use at a co-educational independent school in Toronto, Canada.

OUR RESEARCH

The standardized questionnaire (25) was circulated to Grade 7 through 12 students at Crestwood Preparatory College, an independent co-educational day school in Toronto, Canada. The primary objectives of the survey were to determine 1) the percentage of cyclists at the school and 2) among those cyclists, the percentage who frequently wear a helmet. The questionnaire posed questions regarding bicycle-use on two occasions - the first instance was centred around bicycle-use as a means of transportation to arrive at the school, and the second focused on bicycle-use during recreational time. The secondary objective of the questionnaire was to determine the reasoning or motive of those who do not wear helmets, and subsequently gauge the students' knowledge on legislation around helmet-use. The questionnaire was anonymous, and students were strongly encouraged to complete the survey (25).

The results of the questionnaire were analyzed by grades - Grade 7-8, Grade 9-10 and Grade 11-12. For questions pertaining to frequency of commute and frequency of helmet use, results were collapsed to yield two responses - "Always/Often" and "Rarely/On Occasion/Sometimes." The duration of the commute to school was also divided into two responses - "Under 20 minutes" and "Over 20 minutes." Fisher-exact test was used to examine the difference in proportions for multiple-choice results. Descriptive statistics were used for the short-answer question inquiring about helmet use. All analyses were performed using the Statistical Analysis Software (SAS Version 9.4 for Windows) (25).

WHAT WE FOUND

A total of 77 responses were collected, of which 26 noted that they were in Grade 7-8, 32 in Grade 9-10 and 19 in Grade 11-12. 23%, 22%

and 21% of the cohorts, from youngest to oldest, identified themselves as individuals who cycle to school (p=0.9999). Grade 11-12 students seem to have a shorter commute distance to school than Grade 7 & 8 students (p=0.0858), with 100% as opposed to 50% registering that their commute is under 20 minutes in duration. The same group of students were also more likely to commute to school (p=0.1397; 50% vs 17% for Grade 7-8 students). 50% of Grade 11-12, 43% of Grade 9-10 and 83% of Grade 7-8 students reported that they frequently use a helmet (p=0.4565). 100% of the older students, as opposed to 50% of Grade 7-8 and 29% of Grade 9-10 students were able to identify that there does exist a legislation mandating helmet use (p=0.0858) (see Table 1).

Table 1. Demographics of cyclists to school

	Grades 7 & 8	Grades 9 & 10	Grades 11 & 12	*p*-value
Cyclist/Non-Cyclist				0.9999
Cyclist	6 (23%)	7 (22%)	4 (21%)	
Non-Cyclist	20 (77%)	25 (78%)	15 (79%)	
Duration				0.0858
Under 20 min	3 (50%)	2 (29%)	4 (100%)	
Over 20 min	3 (50%)	5 (71%)	0 (0%)	
Frequency of commute				0.1397
Always/Often	1 (17%)	0 (0%)	2 (50%)	
Rarely/On Occasion/Sometimes	5 (83%)	7 (100%)	2 (50%)	
Frequency of helmet use				0.4565
Always/Often	5 (83%)	3 (43%)	2 (50%)	
Rarely/On Occasion/Sometimes	1 (17%)	4 (57%)	2 (50%)	
Legislation about helmet use				0.0858
True	3 (50%)	2 (29%)	4 (100%)	
False	3 (50%)	5 (71%)	0 (0%)	

92% of Grade 7-8 students reported they were recreational cyclists, while 75% of Grade 9-10 and 68% of Grade 11-12 students similarly reported so (p=0.0971). There was no difference in terms of proportion of students who frequently use a helmet (p=0.9265); 79% of Grade 7-8 students, 71% of Grade 9-10 students and 77% of Grade 11-12 students noted that they regularly use a helmet when cycling. 63%, 79% and 77% of the same groups, respectively, noted that there does exist a legislation around helmet use (p=0.4058) (see Table 2).

Table 2. Demographics of recreational cyclists

	Grades 7 & 8	Grades 9 & 10	Grades 11 & 12	*p*-value
Cyclist/Non-Cyclist				0.0971
Cyclist	24 (92%)	24 (75%)	13 (68%)	
Non-Cyclist	2 (8%)	8 (25%)	6 (32%)	
Frequency of helmet use				0.9265
Always/Often	19 (79%)	17 (71%)	10 (77%)	
Rarely/On Occasion/Sometimes	5 (21%)	7 (29%)	3 (23%)	
Legislation about helmet use				0.4058
True	15 (63%)	19 (79%)	10 (77%)	
False	9 (38%)	5 (21%)	3 (23%)	

Eight reasons were provided by student cyclists; one given by a Grade 7-8 student, five from Grade 9-10 students and two from Grade 11-12 students. The Grade 7-8 student noted that he/she is a safe cyclist and hence does not need a helmet. Two Grade 9-10 students reported that they do not own a helmet, and another two reported that they are a safe cyclist; one student provided another reason. Both Grade 11-12 students recorded that they simply forgot their helmet and hence did not use it regularly (see Table 3).

Table 3. Reasons for not wearing a helmet - school commute

Reasons	Grades 7 & 8	Grades 9 & 10	Grades 11 & 12
Don't have one	0 (0%)	2 (40%)	0 (0%)
I'm a safe cyclist/ Don't consider myself needing one	1 (100%)	2 (40%)	0 (0%)
I forget it	0 (0%)	0 (0%)	2 (100%)
Other*:	0 (0%)	1 (20%)	0 (0%)

*Other: Too bulky, Cannot find it/ In a rush.

Seven excuses were provided by Grade 7-8 recreational cyclists, while seven and four were provided by Grade 9-10, and Grade 11-12 students, respectively. The most commonly cited reason by Grade 7-8 students were their belief they are a safe rider and do not need one (71%), followed by the uncomfortable nature (14%) and inability to find it (14%). In the Grade 9-10 cohort, the most common reason was its uncomfortable nature (57%), with 29% noting other reasons and 14% noting that it is a short trip. Grade 11-12 students equally reported that they are a safe rider (50%) and reported other reasons (50%) (see Table 4).

Table 4. Reasons for not wearing a helmet - recreational cycling

Reasons	Grades 7 & 8	Grades 9 & 10	Grades 11 & 12
It's uncomfortable	1 (14%)	4 (57%)	0 (0%)
I don't want to/ I'm a safe rider/ It's a short trip	5 (71%)	1 (14%)	2 (50%)
Can't find it	1 (14%)	0 (0%)	0 (0%)
Other*:	0 (0%)	2 (29%)	2 (50%)

*Other: Don't have one, Unattractive to wear one, Helmets are useless.

DISCUSSION

This study failed to record a negative correlation between age and bicycle helmet use. This may be a result of different upbringings of adolescents in this population. Additionally, the lack of trend may be a result of a relatively smaller sample size than previous studies. Nevertheless, the results show that a handful of students do not regularly use a helmet, leaving much room for improvement.

The percentage of individuals who are aware of the legislation is lower than the proportion of those who regularly wear a helmet, in general. Given that the percentage of those wearing a helmet is higher, this suggests that students regularly wear a helmet not necessarily due to their abidement to the law but rather for other reasons (i.e., parent encouragement).

In order to improve the frequency of helmet use, educational programs could be employed to increase the awareness of the legislation of helmet use. This could lead to more students being aware of the implications of not wearing a helmet should law enforcement investigate into them, and resultantly a higher percentage of students wearing a helmet. The most common reasons for not wearing a helmet suggest that the educational programs could emphasize that accidents could occur beyond the control of the rider and helmets would ultimately be the best safety equipment.

There seems to exist a trend that a higher proportion of younger adolescents use a bicycle during their recreational time. This may be a result of older students typically having greater workload and decreasing the amount of recreational time, in addition to prioritizing other activities such as meeting up with friends during their free time.

This study has its limitations. The sample size was smaller than some previously conducted and hence has lower statistical power. In addition, due to the nature of the survey methods, there exists the possibility of both a response and sampling bias.

In conclusion, this study suggests that there does not exist a negative correlation with respect to age and helmet use. This may be a result of different upbringings of adolescents in this population. Additionally, the percentage of individuals who are aware of the legislation is lower than the proportion of those who regularly wear a helmet. In order to improve the frequency of helmet use, educational programs could be employed to increase the awareness of the legislation of helmet use. This could lead to more students being aware of the implications of not wearing a helmet should law enforcement investigate into them, and resultantly a higher percentage of students wearing a helmet. The programs could also further emphasize the efficacy of helmets.

Acknowledgments

We would like to thank all of those who participated in the questionnaire.

References

[1]   Chow R, Borean M, Hollenberg D, Ganguli N, Freedman Z, Kang R, et al. Helmet use of young adults in New York State, United States of America. Int J Child Health Hum Dev 2018;11(1), in press.
[2]   Anpalagan T, Hollenberg D, Borean M, Rzepka A, Chow R. Helmet use of young adults in London, Canada. Int J Child Health Hum Dev 2018;11(1), in press.
[3]   Anpalagan T, Panigrahi I, Borean M, Hollenberg D, Rzepka A, Viehweger J et al. Helmet use of young adults in Hamilton, Canada. Int J Child Health Hum Dev 2018;11(1); in press.,
[4]   Rzepka A, Borean M, Hollenberg D, Chan Z, Binns A, Weise E, et al. Helmet use of young adults in Guelph, Canada. Int J Child Health Hum Dev 2018;11(1), in press.
[5]   Anpalagan T, Duarte N, Borean M, Anpalagan J, Camilleri R, Hollenberg D, et al. Helmet use of young adults in Waterloo, Canada. Int J Child Health Hum Dev 2018;11(1), in press.

[6] Chow R, Borean M, Hollenberg D, Ho C, Ng W, Guo W, et al. Helmet use of young adults in Toronto, Canada. Int J Child Health Hum Dev 2018;11(1), in press.

[7] Viehweger J, Borean M, Tang M, Hollenberg D, Anpalagan T, Rzepka A, et al. Helmet use of young adults in St. Catherines, Canada. Int J Child Health Hum Dev 2018;11(1), in press.

[8] Viehweger J, Borean M, Midroni L, Midroni C, Hollenberg D, Anpalagan T et al. Helmet use of young adults in Kingston, Canada. Int J Child Health Hum Dev 2018;11(1), in press.

[9] Chow R, Borean M, Hollenberg D, Song K, Liu J, Young T, et al. Helmet use of young adults in Montreal, Canada. Int J Child Health Hum Dev 2018;11(1), in press.

[10] Chow R, Rzepka A, Borean M, Parekh R, Hollenberg D, Anpalagan T, et al. Helmet use of young adults in Saskatoon, Canada. Int J Child Health Hum Dev 2018;11(1), in press.

[11] Hollenberg D, Ferguson T, Borean M, Anpalagan T, Rzepka A, Viehweger J, et al. Helmet use of young adults in Halifax, Canada. Int J Child Health Hum Dev 2018;11(1), in press.

[12] Chow R, Borean M, Murai A, Menon G, Hollenberg D, Anpalagan T, et al. Helmet use of young adults in California, United States of America. Int J Child Health Hum Dev 2018;11(1), in press.

[13] Chow R, Hollenberg D, Borean M, Goh S, Anpalagan T, Rzepka A, et al. Helmet use of young adults in Dublin, Ireland. Int J Child Health Hum Dev 2018;11(1), in press.

[14] Chow R. Bicycle and helmet use of young adults and adolescents: a meta-analysis. Int J Child Health Hum Dev 2018;11(1), in press.

[15] Chow R, Hollenberg D, Pintilie A, Midroni C, Cumner S. Helmet use of adolescent cyclists at Crescent School in Toronto, Canada. Int J Adolesc Med Health 2016, in press.

[16] Borean M, Ho S, Hollenberg D, Anpalagan T, Rzepka A, Viehweger J, et al. Helmet use of adolescents in Markham, Canada. Int J Adolesc Med Health 2017, in press.

[17] Anpalagan T, Borean M, Chen L, Viehweger J, Hollenberg D, Rzepka A, et al. Helmet use of adolescents in Toronto, Canada. Int J Child Health Hum Dev 2018;11(1), in press.

[18] Borean M, Trasente V, Rzepka A, Viggiani D, Viotto D, Hollenberg D, et al. Helmet use of adolescents at De La Salle Oaklands in Toronto, Canada. Int J Child Health Hum Dev 2018;11(1), in press.

[19] Chow R, Borean M, Hollenberg D, Viehweger J, Young K, Young A et al. Helmet use of adolescents at Ashbury College in Ottawa, Canada. Int J Child Health Hum Dev 2019, in press.

[20] Chow R, Borean M, Hollenberg D, Viehweger J, Hesse J. Helmet use of adolescents at Aberdeen Hall in Kelowna, Canada. Int J Child Health Hum Dev 2019, in press.

[21] Chow R, Borean M, Hollenberg D, Viehweger J, Alexander B, Gladstone J. Helmet use of adolescents at Linden School in Toronto, Canada. Int J Child Health Hum Dev 2019, in press.
[22] Viehweger J, Borean M, Hollenberg D, Cuzzetto S, Chow R. Helmet use of adolescents at Kamloops Christian School in Kamloops, Canada. Int J Child Health Hum Dev 2019, in press.
[23] Chow R, Viehweger J, Borean M, Hollenberg D. Helmet use of adolescents at Avon Old Farms School in Avon, USA. Int J Child Health Hum Dev 2019, in press.
[24] Chow R, Borean M, Hollenberg D, Viehweger J. Helmet use of adolescents at Southridge School in Surrey, Canada. Int J Child Health Hum Dev 2019, in press.
[25] Chow R. Bicycle and helmet use: the survey instrument. Int J Child Health Hum Dev 2019, in press.

In: Bicycles
Editors: Ronald Chow et al.

ISBN: 978-1-53612-458-3
© 2017 Nova Science Publishers, Inc.

Chapter 6

HELMET USE OF ADOLESCENTS AT ELMWOOD SCHOOL IN OTTAWA, CANADA

Ronald Chow[1,]*, BMSc(C),
Michael Borean[1], BMSc(C),
Drew Hollenberg[1], BMSc(C),
Jaclyn Viehweger[1], BMSc(C),
James Whitehouse[2], PGCE,
and Cheryl Boughton[2], BEd

[1]Bicycle Safety and Awareness Club, London, Ontario, Canada
[2]Elmwood School, Ottawa, Ontario, Canada

There seems to exist variation between adolescents in different regions with respect to how often they wear helmets, and hence more studies need to be conducted to look at whether a negative correlation between age and helmet use prevails in these regions. The aim of this chapter was to determine the helmet use rate of adolescents at Elmwood School in

---

* Correspondence: Ronald Chow BMSc(C), Bicycle Safety and Awareness Club, London, Ontario, Canada. Email: rchow48@uwo.ca.

Ottawa, Ontario, Canada. The primary objectives of the circulated survey were to determine 1) the percentage of cyclists at the school and 2) among those cyclists, the percentage who frequently wear a helmet. The questionnaire posed questions regarding bicycle-use on two occasions - the first instance was centred around bicycle-use as a means of transportation to and from the school, and the second focused on bicycle-use during recreational time. The secondary objective of the questionnaire was to determine the reasoning or motive of those who do not wear helmets, and subsequently gauge the students' knowledge on legislation around helmet-use. In conclusion, this is the first study to look into Grade 6 students in addition to Grade 7-12 students. The results show that even with the additional age cohort, the negative correlation previously reported stands. Educational programs can be employed in all groups to hopefully increase helmet wearing by teaching about the safety benefits, as none of the groups have perfect adherence.

INTRODUCTION

Helmet use of young adults is well documented (1-13), with thirteen studies compiled into a meta-analysis to reveal that there exists a positive trend between age and helmet use (14). The studies, which were conducted in different geographical regions, all reported a similar positive correlation but also revealed variation in popularity of helmet use between the regions.

Fewer studies have looked into the helmet use of adolescents (15-24). One could argue that there exists even greater variation in this age cohort as opposed to young adults, as revealed by published studies. Chow et al. reported that 96% of Grade 7 and 8 students regularly use a helmet (15), while a study by Borean et al. at another independent school within close proximity had the statistic at 80% (16).

There seems to exist great variation in this age group, and hence more studies need to be conducted to look at whether a trend prevails in these regions. The aim of this study was to determine the helmet use rate of adolescents at Elmwood School in Ottawa, Ontario, Canada.

OUR STUDY

The standardized questionnaire (25) was circulated to Grade 6 through 12 students at Elmwood School, an independent all-girls day school in Ottawa, Canada. The primary objectives of the survey were to determine 1) the percentage of cyclists at the school and 2) among those cyclists, the percentage who frequently wear a helmet. The questionnaire posed questions regarding bicycle-use on two occasions - the first instance was centred around bicycle-use as a means of transportation to arrive at the school, and the second focused on bicycle-use during recreational time. The secondary objective of the questionnaire was to determine the reasoning or motive of those who do not wear helmets, and subsequently gauge the students' knowledge on legislation around helmet-use. The questionnaire was anonymous, and students were strongly encouraged to complete the survey (25).

The results of the questionnaire were analyzed by grades - Grade 6, Grade 7-8, Grade 9-10 and Grade 11-12. For questions pertaining to frequency of commute and frequency of helmet use, results were collapsed to yield two responses - "Always/Often" and "Rarely/On Occasion/Sometimes." The duration of the commute to school was also divided into two responses - "Under 20 minutes" and "Over 20 minutes." Chi-square tests and Fisher-exact tests was used to examine the difference in proportions for multiple-choice results. Descriptive statistics were used for the short-answer question inquiring about helmet use. All analyses were performed using the Statistical Analysis Software (SAS Version 9.4 for Windows) (25).

FINDINGS

A total of 144 responses were collected, of which 23 students identified themselves as Grade 6 students, 53 noted they were a Grade 7 or 8 student, 36 as Grade 9-10, and 32 as Grade 11-12. A lower percentage of older students remarked that they bike to school (p = 0.0685; 16% compared to 48% for Grade 6 students) and that they frequently do so (p = 0.0959; 60% compared to 73% of Grade 6 students). The majority of students, regardless of grade, do not regularly commute to school via bicycle (p = 0.2639) - 27% of Grade 6, 25% of Grade 7-8, and 0% of Grade 9-12 students regularly bike to school. Statistical analysis did not conclude that older students use helmets less regularly than younger students (p = 0.4700), even though percentages suggested otherwise (60% use among Grade 11-12 students, while the rate was 91% for Grade 6 students). An overwhelming majority of students are aware that there exists legislation mandating helmet use (p = 0.9999) (see Table 1).

A higher percentage of younger students reported that they use their bicycle during their free time (p = 0.0139), with 78% of Grades 11-12 students reporting they are recreational cyclists, 69% of Grades 9-10 similarly reporting so, in addition to 96% of Grades 6-8 students. There was a statistical difference between the age cohorts in the percentage of students who were a helmet regularly (p = 0.0014); 52%, 76%, 88% and 91%, from the oldest to youngest cohort respectively, regularly use a helmet. There was no substantial difference between the age cohorts with respect to knowledge about the legislation (p=0.6674) (see Table 2).

Eight reasons were provided by student cyclists as to why they do not regularly use a helmet - one from Grade 6 students, three from Grade 7-8 students, one from Grade 9-10 students and three from Grade 11-12 students. The Grade 6 student noted that they do not have a helmet. Two Grade 7-8 students noted that it is a short ride and hence did not need a helmet, while the other simply reported the uncomfortable nature of a helmet. The Grade 9-10 student noted uncomfort as the deterrent for not using a helmet regularly. Grades 11-12 students primarily noted that they forgot or do not have a helmet, and that helmets are uncomfortable (see Table 3).

Table 1. Demographics of cyclists to school

	Grade 6	Grades 7 & 8	Grades 9 & 10	Grades 11 & 12	*p*-value
Cyclist/Non-Cyclist					0.0685
Cyclist	11 (48%)	16 (30%)	9 (25%)	5 (16%)	
Non-Cyclist	12 (52%)	37 (70%)	27 (75%)	27 (84%)	
Duration					0.0959
Under 20 min	8 (73%)	15 (94%)	5 (56%)	3 (60%)	
Over 20 min	3 (27%)	1 (6%)	4 (44%)	2 (40%)	
Frequency of commute					0.2639
Always/Often	3 (27%)	4 (25%)	0 (0%)	0 (0%)	
Rarely/On Occasion/Sometimes	8 (73%)	12 (75%)	9 (100%)	5 (100%)	
Frequency of helmet use					0.4700
Always/Often	10 (91%)	12 (75%)	8 (89%)	3 (60%)	
Rarely/On Occasion/Sometimes	1 (9%)	4 (25%)	1 (11%)	2 (40%)	
Legislation about helmet use					0.9999
True	10 (91%)	15 (94%)	9 (100%)	5 (100%)	
False	1 (9%)	1 (6%)	0 (0%)	0 (0%)	

Thirty six excuses were given by recreational cyclists; 4 from Grade 6s, 11 from Grades 7-8, 7 from Grades 9-10, and 14 from Grades 11-12. Grade 6 students equally reported that they do not have a helmet (50%) and that it is a short ride (50%). The majority of Grade 7-8 students gave other reasons (46%), followed by the reason that it is a short ride (27%), they forget (18%) and that they are a safe rider (9%). 43% of Grade 9-10 students noted that it is a short ride and hence does not need a helmet, in addition to other reasons (29%), that they are a safe rider (14%) and that they do not have one (14%). Grade 11-12 students reported that they do not have one (36%), that it is a short ride (21%), that they are a safe rider (14%) and other reasons (29%) (see Table 4).

Table 2. Demographics of recreational cyclists

	Grade 6	Grades 7 & 8	Grades 9 & 10	Grades 11 & 12	*p*-value
Cyclist/Non-Cyclist					0.0139
Cyclist	22 (96%)	51 (96%)	25 (69%)	25 (78%)	
Non-Cyclist	1 (4%)	2 (4%)	11 (31%)	7 (22%)	
Frequency of helmet use					0.0014
Always/Often	20 (91%)	45 (88%)	19 (76%)	13 (52%)	
Rarely/On Occasion/Sometimes	2 (9%)	6 (12%)	6 (24%)	12 (48%)	
Legislation about helmet use					0.6674
True	21 (95%)	45 (88%)	22 (88%)	21 (84%)	
False	1 (5%)	6 (12%)	3 (12%)	4 (16%)	

Table 3. Reasons for not wearing a helmet - school commute

Reasons	Grade 6	Grades 7 & 8	Grades 9 & 10	Grades 11 & 12
I am a safe rider/It's a short ride	0 (0%)	2 (67%)	0 (0%)	0 (0%)
Helmets are uncomfortable	0 (0%)	1 (33%)	1 (100%)	1 (67%)
Don't have one/I forget	1 (100%)	0 (0%)	0 (0%)	2 (33%)

Table 4. Reasons for not wearing a helmet - recreational cycling

Reasons	Grade 6	Grades 7 & 8	Grades 9 & 10	Grades 11 & 12
Don't have one/I forget	2 (50%)	2 (18%)	1 (14%)	5 (36%)
It's a short ride/I'm being supervised	2 (50%)	3 (27%)	3 (43%)	3 (21%)
I'm a safe rider	0 (0%)	1 (9%)	1 (14%)	2 (14%)
Other*:	0 (0%)	5 (46%)	2 (29%)	4 (29%)

* Other: Inconvenient/ Uncomfortable, Doesn't fit, Helmets are useless.

DISCUSSION

The results contained herein revealed that there exists a negative correlation between age and helmet use in the studied population. This study is the first to look at Grade 6 students, in addition to Grade 7-12 students, and shows that even with the additional age cohort, the negative correlation previously reported stands.

The results also show that older students do not use a helmet as regularly as younger students, in both the school commute setting and the recreational setting. This may be a result of older children using other means of transportation to school (i.e., public transit, driving their own car), and also using their recreational time in other activities (i.e., going with friends to movies, participating in gatherings).

In the two youngest age cohorts, the proportion of students who are aware of the legislation and who regularly use a helmet are approximately equal, suggesting that students use a helmet as a result of the knowledge of legislation. In the older groups, the percentage of knowledge of legislation is higher than the other statistic, which may suggest that lack of helmet use is a result of a lack of desire to adhere to established legislation. Educational programs can be employed in all groups to hopefully increase helmet wearing by teaching about the safety benefits, as none of the groups have perfect adherence.

This study was not without limitations. As with any survey study, there exists the possibility of a sample and response bias. This was hopefully mitigated by the sample size, which would normalize the data to a certain extent.

In conclusion, this is the first study to look into Grade 6 students in addition to Grade 7-12 students. The results show that even with the additional age cohort, the negative correlation previously reported stands. Educational programs can be employed in all groups to hopefully increase helmet wearing by teaching about the safety benefits, as none of the groups have perfect adherence.

ACKNOWLEDGMENTS

We would like to thank all of those who participated in the questionnaire.

REFERENCES

[1] Chow R, Borean M, Hollenberg D, Ganguli N, Freedman Z, Kang R, et al. Helmet use of young adults in New York State, United States of America. Int J Child Health Hum Dev 2018;11(1), in press.
[2] Anpalagan T, Hollenberg D, Borean M, Rzepka A, Chow R. Helmet use of young adults in London, Canada. Int J Child Health Hum Dev 2018;11(1), in press.
[3] Anpalagan T, Panigrahi I, Borean M, Hollenberg D, Rzepka A, Viehweger J et al. Helmet use of young adults in Hamilton, Canada. Int J Child Health Hum Dev 2018;11(1), in press.
[4] Rzepka A, Borean M, Hollenberg D, Chan Z, Binns A, Weise E, et al. Helmet use of young adults in Guelph, Canada. Int J Child Health Hum Dev 2018;11(1), in press.
[5] Anpalagan T, Duarte N, Borean M, Anpalagan J, Camilleri R, Hollenberg D, et al. Helmet use of young adults in Waterloo, Canada. Int J Child Health Hum Dev 2018;11(1), in press.
[6] Chow R, Borean M, Hollenberg D, Ho C, Ng W, Guo W, et al. Helmet use of young adults in Toronto, Canada. Int J Child Health Hum Dev 2018;11(1), in press.
[7] Viehweger J, Borean M, Tang M, Hollenberg D, Anpalagan T, Rzepka A, et al. Helmet use of young adults in St. Catherines, Canada. Int J Child Health Hum Dev 2018;11(1), in press.
[8] Viehweger J, Borean M, Midroni L, Midroni C, Hollenberg D, Anpalagan T et al. Helmet use of young adults in Kingston, Canada. Int J Child Health Hum Dev 2018;11(1), in press.
[9] Chow R, Borean M, Hollenberg D, Song K, Liu J, Young T, et al. Helmet use of young adults in Montreal, Canada. Int J Child Health Hum Dev 2018;11(1), in press.
[10] Chow R, Rzepka A, Borean M, Parekh R, Hollenberg D, Anpalagan T, et al. Helmet use of young adults in Saskatoon, Canada. Int J Child Health Hum Dev 2018;11(1), in press.
[11] Hollenberg D, Ferguson T, Borean M, Anpalagan T, Rzepka A, Viehweger J, et al. Helmet use of young adults in Halifax, Canada. Int J Child Health Hum Dev 2018;11(1), in press.

[12] Chow R, Borean M, Murai A, Menon G, Hollenberg D, Anpalagan T, et al. Helmet use of young adults in California, United States of America. Int J Child Health Hum Dev 2018;11(1), in press.

[13] Chow R, Hollenberg D, Borean M, Goh S, Anpalagan T, Rzepka A, et al. Helmet use of young adults in Dublin, Ireland. Int J Child Health Hum Dev 2018;11(1), in press.

[14] Chow R. Bicycle and helmet use of young adults and adolescents: A meta-analysis. Int J Child Health Hum Dev 2018;11(1), in press.

[15] Chow R, Hollenberg D, Pintilie A, Midroni C, Cumner S. Helmet use of adolescent cyclists at Crescent School in Toronto, Canada. Int J Adolesc Med Health 2016, in press.

[16] Borean M, Ho S, Hollenberg D, Anpalagan T, Rzepka A, Viehweger J, et al. Helmet use of adolescents in Markham, Canada. Int J Adolesc Med Health 2017, in press.

[17] Anpalagan T, Borean M, Chen L, Viehweger J, Hollenberg D, Rzepka A, et al. Helmet use of adolescents in Toronto, Canada. Int J Child Health Hum Dev 2018;11(1), in press.

[18] Borean M, Trasente V, Rzepka A, Viggiani D, Viotto D, Hollenberg D, et al. Helmet use of adolescents at De La Salle Oaklands in Toronto, Canada. Int J Child Health Hum Dev 2018;11(1), in press.

[19] Chow R, Borean M, Hollenberg D, Viehweger J, Young K, Young A et al. Helmet use of adolescents at Ashbury College in Ottawa, Canada. Int J Child Health Hum Dev 2019, in press.

[20] Chow R, Borean M, Hollenberg D, Viehweger J, Hesse J. Helmet use of adolescents at Aberdeen Hall in Kelowna, Canada. Int J Child Health Hum Dev 2019, in press.

[21] Chow R, Borean M, Hollenberg D, Viehweger J, Alexander B, Gladstone J. Helmet use of adolescents at Linden School in Toronto, Canada. Int J Child Health Hum Dev 2019, in press.

[22] Viehweger J, Borean M, Hollenberg D, Cuzzetto S, Chow R. Helmet use of adolescents at Kamloops Christian School in Kamloops, Canada. Int J Child Health Hum Dev 2019, in press.

[23] Chow R, Viehweger J, Borean M, Hollenberg D. Helmet use of adolescents at Avon Old Farms School in Avon, USA. Int J Child Health Hum Dev 2019, in press.

[24] Chow R, Borean M, Hollenberg D, Viehweger J, Smith B. Helmet use of adolescents at Southridge School in Surrey, Canada. Int J Child Health Hum Dev 2019, in press.

[25] Chow R. Bicycle and helmet use: the survey instrument. Int J Child Health Hum Dev 2019, in press.

Section three: British Columbia

In: Bicycles
Editors: Ronald Chow et al.

ISBN: 978-1-53612-458-3
© 2017 Nova Science Publishers, Inc.

Chapter 7

HELMET USE OF ADOLESCENTS AT ABERDEEN HALL IN KELOWNA, CANADA

Ronald Chow[1,*], BMSc(C), Michael Borean[1], BMSc(C), Drew Hollenberg[1], BMSc(C), Jaclyn Viehweger[1], BMSc(C) and Jerry Hesse[2], BEd

[1]Bicycle Safety and Awareness Club, London, Ontario, Canada
[2]Aberdeen Hall Preparatory School, Kelowna, British Columbia, Canada

When comparing the helmet use rates of secondary schools in Toronto and Ottawa, there exists variation in the helmet-use rates and variation in frequency of cycling. It seems that different geographical regions have adolescents with different biking practices. The aim of this chapter was to investigate the biking practices of adolescents in Kelowna, British Columbia, Canada. The primary objectives of the survey were to determine 1) the percentage of cyclists at the school and 2) among those cyclists, the percentage who frequently wear a helmet. The secondary

---

[*] Correspondence: Ronald Chow BMSc(C), Bicycle Safety and Awareness Club, London, Ontario, Canada. Email: rchow48@uwo.ca.

objective of the questionnaire was to determine the reasoning or motive of those who do not wear helmets, and subsequently gauge the students' knowledge on legislation around helmet-use. The questionnaire was anonymous, and students were strongly encouraged during school-allotted time to complete the survey. This study suggests that there does not exist a negative correlation with respect to age and helmet use, among the adolescent population in Kelowna, British Columbia, Canada. However, the small sample size limited statistical power and hence results should be interpreted with caution. Follow-up studies should be carried out before any action were to be taken in response to the results contained herein. Nevertheless, the data does show that there is room for improvement with respect to helmet-use; educational/encouragement programs could be designed to hopefully encourage more regular helmet-use.

INTRODUCTION

A meta-analysis conducted by Chow revealed that there is a U-shaped relationship between age and helmet-use, among adolescents and young adults. The seventeen studies included in the review suggested that young adolescents most often use a helmet, with the proportion of individuals using such a safety device when cycling decreasing as adolescents age, but eventually increasing again as young adults age (1).

Five studies (2-6) have thus far looked into the suggested negative correlation by Chow et al. (2). The first study was conducted at Crescent School, an independent all-boys day school in Toronto, Canada. Grade 7 and 8 students were reported to use helmets 96% of the time, Grade 9 and 10 students 76% of the time, and Grade 11 and 12 students 59% of the time. This negative correlation was validated in subsequent studies at other schools in Toronto (3-5) and Ottawa (6).

When comparing the helmet use rates of secondary schools in Toronto and Ottawa, there exists variation in the helmet-use rates and variation in frequency of cycling. It seems that different geographical regions have adolescents with different biking practices. The aim of this study was to investigate the biking practices of adolescents in Kelowna, British Columbia, Canada.

OUR STUDY

The questionnaire was circulated to Grade 7 through 12 students at Aberdeen Hall Preparatory School, an independent co-educational day school in Kelowna, Canada. The primary objectives of the survey were to determine 1) the percentage of cyclists at the school and 2) among those cyclists, the percentage who frequently wear a helmet. The questionnaire posed questions regarding bicycle-use on two occasions - the first instance was centred around bicycle-use as a means of transportation to arrive at the school, and the second focused on bicycle-use during recreational time. The secondary objective of the questionnaire was to determine the reasoning or motive of those who do not wear helmets, and subsequently gauge the students' knowledge on legislation around helmet-use. The questionnaire was anonymous, and students were strongly encouraged to complete the survey (7).

The results of the questionnaire were analyzed by grades - Grade 7 and 8, Grade 9 and 10, Grade 11 and 12. For questions pertaining to frequency of commute and frequency of helmet use, results were collapsed to yield two responses - "Always/Often" and "Rarely/On Occasion/Sometimes". The duration of the commute to school was also divided into two responses - "Under 20 minutes" and "Over 20 minutes". Fisher-exact test was used to examine the difference in proportions for multiple-choice results. Descriptive statistics were used for the short-answer question inquiring about helmet use. All analyses were performed using the Statistical Analysis Software (SAS Version 9.4 for Windows) (7).

FINDINGS

A total of 34 students completed the questionnaire; 9 were Grade 7 and 8 students, 14 were in Grade 9 and 10, and 11 were in Grade 11 and 12. No Grade 7 and 8 students (0%), 1 Grade 9 and 10 (7%), and 1 Grade 11 and 12 (9%) student identified themselves as a cyclist who commutes to school (p = 0.9999). Both student cyclists remarked that their commute takes under 20 minutes (p = 0.9999) and that they do not frequently bike to school (p = 0.9999). Both do not regularly wear a helmet when they do commute (p = 0.9999). The younger student (Grade 9 and 10) was aware that there exists a legislation mandating helmet use, while the older student (Grade 11 and 12) was not aware of the mandate (p = 0.9999) (see Table 1).

Table 1. Demographics of cyclists to school

	Grades 7 & 8	Grades 9 & 10	Grades 11 & 12	p-value
Cyclist/Non-Cyclist				0.9999
Cyclist	0 (0%)	1 (7%)	1 (9%)	
Non-Cyclist	9 (100%)	13 (93%)	10 (91%)	
Duration				0.9999
Under 20 min	0 (0%)	1 (100%)	1 (100%)	
Over 20 min	0 (0%)	0 (0%)	0 (0%)	
Frequency of commute				0.9999
Always/Often	0 (0%)	0 (0%)	0 (0%)	
Rarely/On Occasion/Sometimes	0 (0%)	1 (100%)	1 (100%)	
Frequency of helmet use				0.9999
Always/Often	0 (0%)	0 (0%)	0 (0%)	
Rarely/On Occasion/Sometimes	0 (0%)	1 (100%)	1 (100%)	
Legislation about helmet use				0.9999
True	0 (0%)	1 (100%)	0 (0%)	
False	0 (0%)	0 (0%)	1 (100%)	

Table 2. Demographics of recreational cyclists

	Grades 7 & 8	Grades 9 & 10	Grades 11 & 12	*p*-value
Cyclist/Non-Cyclist				0.8057
Cyclist	8 (89%)	13 (93%)	9 (82%)	
Non-Cyclist	1 (11%)	1 (7%)	2 (18%)	
Frequency of helmet use				0.1777
Always/Often	7 (88%)	7 (54%)	8 (89%)	
Rarely/On Occasion/Sometimes	1 (12%)	6 (46%)	1 (11%)	
Legislation about helmet use				0.4842
True	5 (62%)	11 (85%)	7 (78%)	
False	3 (38%)	2 (15%)	2 (22%)	

The majority of students reported that they are recreational cyclists; 89% of the youngest, 93% of the middle-aged and 82% of the oldest cohort noted that they use their bicycle during their recreational time (p = 0.8057). Grade 9 and 10 students seem to not wear helmets as regularly (54%) as Grade 7 and 8 (88%), and Grade 11 and 12 (89%) students (p = 0.1777). There was no difference in knowledge level about the helmet legislation (p = 0.4842) - 62% of Grade 7 and 8, 85% of Grade 9 and 10, and 78% of Grade 11 and 12 students remarked that there does exist a law and that they are aware of it (p = 0.4842) (see Table 2).

Only one of the two school commuters provided a reason for not using a helmet - it is inconvenient (100%) (see Table 3). Seven reasons were provided by recreational cyclists - three by Grade 7 and 8, two by Grade 9 and 10, and two by Grade 11 and 12 students. Two students (66%) of the youngest group noted that they commute short distances and hence do not need a helmet, while the remaining one (33%) noted that helmets are uncomfortable. One Grade 9 and 10 student (50%) similarly noted the short trip, and the other (50%) reported that they do not own a helmet. Both students in Grade 11 and 12 (100%) reported that their recreational commutes are short trips and do not necessitate a helmet.

Table 3. Reasons for not wearing a helmet - school commute

Reasons	Grades 7 & 8	Grades 9 & 10	Grades 11 & 12
Helmets are inconvenient	0 (0%)	1 (100%)	0 (0%)

DISCUSSION

While previous studies (2-5) suggested a negative correlation between helmet use and age, this study does not detect a negative correlation. This could perhaps be explained by different upbringings of adolescents which foster a different environment around helmet use. This lack of trend may also be a result of a small sample size, which reduces the statistical power. The results do show that not all students regularly use a helmet though, still suggesting that there may be room for change.

The study also suggests that while a large proportion of recreational cyclists use their helmets during their recreational time. The reported frequency is noticeably higher than other studies (2-6), and may also be a result of different childhood and adolescent developments as a result of different geographical region and consequently environment. However, this too should be interpreted with caution due to the sample size.

When comparing the frequency of helmet use and the knowledge of legislation, the rate of frequent helmet use seems to be higher than the knowledge level of legislation. This may suggest further that adolescents in this region more often use a helmet out of interest in their safety rather than in an interest to abide the law. This too could be a result of different environmental factors in this region that fosters greater care for health and well-being than studies conducted elsewhere (2-6).

This study was not without limitations. The sample size was small and hence did not lead to high statistical power - results contained herein should be interpreted with great caution, and follow-up studies should be carried out before any action were to be taken in response to the disclosed results. Additionally, due to the nature of the survey methods, there exists the possibility of both a response and sampling bias.

In conclusion, this study suggests that there does not exist a negative correlation with respect to age and helmet use, among the adolescent population in Kelowna, British Columbia, Canada. However, the small sample size limited statistical power and hence results should be interpreted with caution. Follow-up studies should be carried out before any action were to be taken in response to the results contained herein. Nevertheless, the data does show that there is room for improvement with respect to helmet-use; educational/ encouragement programs could be designed to hopefully encourage more regular helmet-use.

Table 4. Reasons for not wearing a helmet - recreational cycling

Reasons	Grades 7 & 8	Grades 9 & 10	Grades 11 & 12
Short trip and don't need a helmet	2 (67%)	1 (50%)	2 (100%)
Helmets are uncomfortable	1 (33%)	0 (0%)	0 (0%)
I don't own one	0 (0%)	1 (50%)	0 (0%)

ACKNOWLEDGMENTS

We would like to thank all of those who participated in the questionnaire.

REFERENCES

[1] Chow R. Bicycle and helmet use of young adults and adolescents: a meta-analysis. Int J Child Health Hum Dev 2018;11(1), in press.
[2] Chow R, Hollenberg D, Pintilie A, Midroni C, Cumner S. Helmet use of adolescent cyclists at Crescent School in Toronto, Canada. Int J Adolesc Med Health 2016, in press.
[3] Borean M, Ho S, Hollenberg D, Anpalagan T, Rzepka A, Viehweger J, et al. Helmet use of adolescents in Markham, Canada. Int J Adolesc Med Health 2017, in press.
[4] Anpalagan T, Borean M, Chen L, Viehweger J, Hollenberg D, Rzepka A, et al. Helmet use of adolescents in Toronto, Canada. Int J Child Health Hum Dev 2018;11(1), in press.
[5] Borean M, Trasente V, Rzepka A, Viggiani D, Viotto D, Hollenberg D, et al. Helmet use of adolescents at De La Salle Oaklands in Toronto, Canada. Int J Child Health Hum Dev 2018;11(1), in press.
[6] Chow R, Borean M, Hollenberg D, Viehweger J, Young K, Southward N. Helmet use of adolescents at Ashbury College in Ottawa, Canada. Int J Child Health Hum Dev 2019, in press.
[7] Chow R. Bicycle and helmet use: the survey instrument. Int J Child Health Hum Dev 2019, in press.

In: Bicycles
Editors: Ronald Chow et al.

ISBN: 978-1-53612-458-3
© 2017 Nova Science Publishers, Inc.

Chapter 8

HELMET USE OF ADOLESCENTS AT SOUTHRIDGE SCHOOL IN SURREY, CANADA

Ronald Chow[1,]*, BMSc(C), Michael Borean[1], BMSc(C), Drew Hollenberg[1], BMSc(C) and Jaclyn Viehweger[1], BMSc(C)
[1]Bicycle Safety and Awareness Club, London, Ontario, Canada

Helmets have been shown to be efficacious in preventing head trauma but a meta-analysis suggests that adoption rates of helmets are not high nor equivalent across different age groups. There also exists considerable variation in helmet wearing rate among adolescents in different geographic regions. The aim of this investigation was to study the helmet wearing rate of adolescents at an independent school in Surrey, British Columbia, Canada. A survey was circulated to Grade 7 to 12 students at Southridge School in Surrey, Canada. The results of the questionnaire were analyzed by grades - Grade 7 and 8, Grade 9 and 10 and Grade 11 and 12. Of the 226 students who completed the survey, 58 identified as Grade 7 and 8 students, 86 noted they were in Grade 9 and 10, while 82

---

* Correspondence: Ronald Chow BMSc(C), Bicycle Safety and Awareness Club, London, Ontario, Canada. Email: rchow48@uwo.ca.

reported they were in Grade 11 and 12. The results suggest that there does not exist a negative correlation with respect to age and helmet use. This may reflect a different upbringing of adolescents in Surrey, British Columbia. Nevertheless, educational/encouragement programs could be designed to hopefully encourage more regular helmet-use.

INTRODUCTION

Helmets have been shown to be efficacious in preventing head trauma (1) but a meta-analysis suggests that adoption rates of helmets are not high nor equivalent across different age groups (2). Based on studies published among the adolescent (3-6) and young adults (7-19), there seems to exist a U-shaped trend between age and helmet use; helmet use decreases as adolescents age and then increase as young adults mature.

While many studies have documented the variation of young adults across the world, fewer has examined the variation of adolescents. Four studies were included in the meta-analysis. Chow et al. noted that frequent helmet use fell from 96% to 59% among adolescent boys (3), while Borean et al. similarly noted a decline, from 88% to 58% (4). The other two studies similarly suggested the negative correlation trend, as with more recent studies that studied the adolescent population (20-24).

Even with the trend seemingly verified, there exists considerable variation in helmet wearing rate among adolescents in different geographic regions. The aim of this study was to study the helmet wearing rate of adolescents at an independent school in Surrey, British Columbia, Canada.

OUR STUDY

The questionnaire was circulated to Grade 7 through 12 students at Southridge School, an independent co-educational day school in Surrey,

Canada (25). The primary objectives of the survey were to determine (1) the percentage of cyclists at the school and (2) among those cyclists, the percentage who frequently wear a helmet. The questionnaire posed questions regarding bicycle-use on two occasions - the first instance was centred around bicycle-use as a means of transportation to arrive at the school, and the second focused on bicycle-use during recreational time. The secondary objective of the questionnaire was to determine the reasoning or motive of those who do not wear helmets, and subsequently gauge the students' knowledge on legislation around helmet-use. The questionnaire was anonymous, and students were strongly encouraged to complete the survey (25).

The results of the questionnaire were analyzed by grades - Grade 7 and 8, Grade 9 and 10, Grade 11 and 12. For questions pertaining to frequency of commute and frequency of helmet use, results were collapsed to yield two responses - "Always/Often" and "Rarely/On Occasion/Sometimes". The duration of the commute to school was also divided into two responses - "Under 20 minutes" and "Over 20 minutes". Fisher-exact test was used to examine the difference in proportions for multiple-choice results. Descriptive statistics were used for the short-answer question inquiring about helmet use. All analyses were performed using the Statistical Analysis Software (SAS Version 9.4 for Windows) (25).

FINDINGS

226 students completed the survey. Of these 226 students, 58 identified as Grade 7 and 8 students, 86 noted they were in Grade 9 and 10, while 82 reported they were in Grade 11 and 12. 19%, 15% and 18% of the cohorts, from youngest to oldest, respectively, reported that they bike to school ($p = 0.8131$). There was no difference in the proportion of cyclists who report that they have a commute time of under 20 minutes to school ($p = 0.2960$); 64% of Grade 7 and 8 students, 62% of Grade 9

and 10, 87% of Grade 11 and 12 noted that they have a short commute time. The majority of students, regardless of age, do not regularly commute to school (p = 0.7423); specifically, 9%, 23% and 13% of the three groups from youngest to oldest do not regularly commute. Statistical analyses did not reveal a different in helmet use between the cohorts (p = 0.9999), yet there exists a noticeable difference with respect to knowledge of helmet legislation (p = 0.0138) (27% for Grade 11 and 12 students, compared to 82% for Grade 7 and 8 students) (see Table 1).

Table 1. Demographics of cyclists to school

	Grades 7 & 8	Grades 9 & 10	Grades 11 & 12	p-value
Cyclist/Non-Cyclist				0.8131
Cyclist	11 (19%)	13 (15%)	15 (18%)	
Non-Cyclist	47 (81%)	73 (85%)	67 (82%)	
Duration				0.2960
Under 20 min	7 (64%)	8 (62%)	13 (87%)	
Over 20 min	4 (36%)	5 (38%)	2 (13%)	
Frequency of commute				0.7423
Always/Often	1 (9%)	3 (23%)	2 (13%)	
Rarely/On Occasion/Sometimes	10 (91%)	10 (77%)	13 (87%)	
Frequency of helmet use				0.9999
Always/Often	5 (45%)	7 (54%)	8 (53%)	
Rarely/On Occasion/Sometimes	6 (55%)	6 (46%)	7 (47%)	
Legislation about helmet use				0.0138
True	9 (82%)	9 (69%)	4 (27%)	
False	2 (18%)	4 (31%)	11 (73%)	

Table 2. Demographics of recreational cyclists

	Grades 7 & 8	Grades 9 & 10	Grades 11 & 12	*p*-value
Cyclist/Non-Cyclist				0.0747
Cyclist	48 (83%)	68 (79%)	55 (67%)	
Non-Cyclist	10 (17%)	18 (21%)	27 (33%)	
Frequency of helmet use				0.9781
Always/Often	32 (67%)	46 (68%)	38 (69%)	
Rarely/On Occasion/Sometimes	16 (33%)	22 (32%)	17 (31%)	
Legislation about helmet use				0.6334
True	43 (90%)	57 (84%)	46 (84%)	
False	5 (10%)	11 (16%)	9 (16%)	

Older students seem to bike less frequently during their recreational time (p = 0.0747), with 67%, 79% and 83% of the student groups, from oldest to youngest respectively, report themselves as recreational cyclists. There exists no difference in the proportion of students who frequently use a helmet (p = 0.9781) and with respect to education about the helmet legislation (p = 0.6334) (see Table 2).

7, 6 and 6 reasons were provided by student cyclists in Grade 7-8, Grade 9-10, and Grade 11-12 students, respectively, for why they do not regularly wear a helmet. Grade 7-8 students frequently reported that they were too lazy or that helmets were uncomfortable (29%), followed by the ugly nature of helmets (14%), they bike a short distance (14%) and other reasons (43%). Grade 9-10 students equally reasoned that helmets are ugly, they commute a short distance or they are a good rider, and other reasons (33% each). The most common reasons for Grade 11-12 students were the uncomfortable nature of helmets (33%) and that students believe they are a good rider (33%), followed by the ugly nature (17%) and other reasons (17%) (see Table 3).

Table 3. Reasons for not wearing a helmet - school commute

Reasons	Grades 7 & 8	Grades 9 & 10	Grades 11 & 12
It is uncomfortable/too lazy to	2 (29%)	0 (0%)	2 (33%)
It is ugly	1 (14%)	2 (33%)	1 (17%)
It is a short ride/I am a good rider	1 (14%)	2 (33%)	2 (33%)
Other*:	3 (43%)	2 (33%)	1 (17%)

* Other: "Do not feel like it", "I do not own one", "Cannot find it".

20, 29 and 16 reasons were provided by recreational cyclists, from youngest to older cohort. 40% of Grade 7-8 students noted that helmets are uncomfortable, while 30%, 15% and 15%, respectively, noted that they are a good rider, helmets are ugly and other reasons. The most common reasons provided by Grade 9-10 students were that the commute distance was short (28%) and other reasons (28%), followed by the ugly nature of helmets (24%) and the uncomfortable nature (21%). Grade 11-12 students equally reasoned that helmets are uncomfortable and they ride a short distance (38% for both), and also that helmets are ugly and other reasons (13% for both) (see table 4).

Table 4. Reasons for not wearing a helmet - recreational cycling

Reasons	Grades 7 & 8	Grades 9 & 10	Grades 11 & 12
It is uncomfortable/too lazy to	8 (40%)	6 (21%)	6 (38%)
It is ugly	3 (15%)	7 (24%)	2 (13%)
It is a short ride/I am a good rider	6 (30%)	8 (28%)	6 (38%)
Other*:	3 (15%)	8 (28%)	2 (13%)

* Other: "Cannot find it", "Inconvenient", "Looks weird".

DISCUSSION

While previous studies (3-6, 20, 22-24) suggested a negative correlation between helmet use and age, this study does not detect a negative correlation. These results are similar to those found among adolescents at Aberdeen Hall (21). These conclusions could be explained by different upbringings of adolescents which foster a different environment around helmet use.

Interestingly, although there exists no difference in the proportion of individuals who wear a helmet regularly, there is a difference in awareness of legislation. The older groups, who wear helmets at equal frequency when compared to the younger groups, are less aware of the legislation. These students may hence wear helmets at the same rate out of personal safety interest or perhaps due to ingrained habits from their childhood. The latter reason further supports the strong environmental factors on the development of adolescents and hence could explain the anomaly of lack of negative correlation between age and helmet use.

The helmet use among student cyclists is lower than recreational cyclists. This could perhaps be mitigated by educational programs offered by the school surrounding helmet safety and encouragement by the school, when cyclists arrive on campus, to encourage helmet use. The helmet use in both the school commute and recreational setting is documented within this adolescent population is still similar to those previously studied - there still exists a significant handful of students who do not regularly wear a helmet. Educational programs could be employed to increase the awareness of legislation and also emphasize the safety benefits of helmets, to hopefully increase the proportion of students who regularly wear a helmet when cycling in both settings.

This study was not without limitations. As a result of the nature of the survey methods, there exists the possibility of both a response and sampling bias. This was mitigated as much as possible by emphasizing that the survey was anonymous in nature, and also by recruiting a substantial sample size to hopefully normalize any odd (anomalous) findings.

In conclusion, this study suggests that there does not exist a negative correlation with respect to age and helmet use. This may reflect a different upbringings of adolescents in Surrey, British Columbia. Nevertheless, educational/encouragement programs could be designed to hopefully encourage more regular helmet-use.

ACKNOWLEDGMENTS

We would like to thank all of those who participated in the questionnaire.

REFERENCES

[1] Attewell RG, Glase K, McFadden M. Bicycle helmet efficacy: a meta-analysis. Accid Anal Prev 2001;33(3):345-52.
[2] Chow R. Bicycle and helmet use of young adults and adolescents: a meta-analysis. Int J Child Health Hum Dev 2018;11(1), in press.
[3] Chow R, Hollenberg D, Pintilie A, Midroni C, Cumner S. Helmet use of adolescent cyclists at Crescent School in Toronto, Canada. Int J Adolesc Med Health 2016, in press.
[4] Borean M, Ho S, Hollenberg D, Anpalagan T, Rzepka A, Viehweger J, et al. Helmet use of adolescents in Markham, Canada. Int J Adolesc Med Health 2017, in press.
[5] Anpalagan T, Borean M, Chen L, Viehweger J, Hollenberg D, Rzepka A, et al. Helmet use of adolescents in Toronto, Canada. Int J Child Health Hum Dev 2018;11(1), in press.
[6] Borean M, Trasente V, Rzepka A, Viggiani D, Viotto D, Hollenberg D, et al. Helmet use of adolescents at De La Salle Oaklands in Toronto, Canada. Int J Child Health Hum Dev 2018;11(1), in press.
[7] Chow R, Borean M, Hollenberg D, Ganguli N, Freedman Z, Kang R, et al. Helmet use of young adults in New York State, United States of America. Int J Child Health Hum Dev 2018;11(1), in press.
[8] Anpalagan T, Hollenberg D, Borean M, Rzepka A, Chow R. Helmet use of young adults in London, Canada. Int J Child Health Hum Dev 2018;11(1), in press.

[9] Anpalagan T, Panigrahi I, Borean M, Hollenberg D, Rzepka A, Viehweger J et al. Helmet use of young adults in Hamilton, Canada. Int J Child Health Hum Dev 2018;11(1), in press.
[10] Rzepka A, Borean M, Hollenberg D, Chan Z, Binns A, Weise E, et al. Helmet use of young adults in Guelph, Canada. Int J Child Health Hum Dev 2018;11(1), in press.
[11] Anpalagan T, Duarte N, Borean M, Anpalagan J, Camilleri R, Hollenberg D, et al. Helmet use of young adults in Waterloo, Canada. Int J Child Health Hum Dev 2018;11(1), in press.
[12] Chow R, Borean M, Hollenberg D, Ho C, Ng W, Guo W, et al. Helmet use of young adults in Toronto, Canada. Int J Child Health Hum Dev 2018;11(1), in press.
[13] Viehweger J, Borean M, Tang M, Hollenberg D, Anpalagan T, Rzepka A, et al. Helmet use of young adults in St. Catherines, Canada. Int J Child Health Hum Dev 2018;11(1), in press.
[14] Viehweger J, Borean M, Midroni L, Midroni C, Hollenberg D, Anpalagan T et al. Helmet use of young adults in Kingston, Canada. Int J Child Health Hum Dev 2018;11(1), in press.
[15] Chow R, Borean M, Hollenberg D, Song K, Liu J, Young T, et al. Helmet use of young adults in Montreal, Canada. Int J Child Health Hum Dev 2018;11(1), in press.
[16] Chow R, Rzepka A, Borean M, Parekh R, Hollenberg D, Anpalagan T, et al. Helmet use of young adults in Saskatoon, Canada. Int J Child Health Hum Dev 2018;11(1), in press.
[17] Hollenberg D, Ferguson T, Borean M, Anpalagan T, Rzepka A, Viehweger J, et al. Helmet use of young adults in Halifax, Canada. Int J Child Health Hum Dev 2018;11(1), in press.
[18] Chow R, Borean M, Murai A, Menon G, Hollenberg D, Anpalagan T, et al. Helmet use of young adults in California, United States of America. Int J Child Health Hum Dev 2018;11(1), in press.
[19] Chow R, Hollenberg D, Borean M, Goh S, Anpalagan T, Rzepka A, et al. Helmet use of young adults in Dublin, Ireland. Int J Child Health Hum Dev 2018;11(1), in press.
[20] Chow R, Borean M, Hollenberg D, Viehweger J, Young K, Young A et al. Helmet use of adolescents at Ashbury College in Ottawa, Canada. Int J Child Health Hum Dev 2019, in press.
[21] Chow R, Borean M, Hollenberg D, Viehweger J, Hesse J. Helmet use of adolescents at Aberdeen Hall in Kelowna, Canada. Int J Child Health Hum Dev 2019, in press.
[22] Chow R, Borean M, Hollenberg D, Viehweger J, Alexander B, Gladstone J. Helmet use of adolescents at Linden School in Toronto, Canada. Int J Child Health Hum Dev 2019; in press.
[23] Viehweger J, Borean M, Hollenberg D, Cuzzetto S, Chow R. Helmet use of adolescents at Kamloops Christian School in Kamloops, Canada. Int J Child Health Hum Dev 2019, in press.

[24] Chow R, Viehweger J, Borean M, Hollenberg D. Helmet use of adolescents at Avon Old Farms School in Avon, USA. Int J Child Health Hum Dev 2019, in press.
[25] Chow R. Bicycle and helmet use: the survey instrument. Int J Child Health Hum Dev 2019, in press.

In: Bicycles
Editors: Ronald Chow et al.

ISBN: 978-1-53612-458-3
© 2017 Nova Science Publishers, Inc.

Chapter 9

HELMET USE OF ADOLESCENTS IN THE PROVINCE OF BRITISH COLUMBIA, CANADA

Jaclyn Viehweger[1],*, BMSc(C),
Michael Borean[1], BMSc(C),
Drew Hollenberg[1], BMSc(C),
Sandro Cuzzetto[2], MEd
and Ronald Chow[1], BMSc(C)

[1]Bicycle Safety and Awareness Club, London, Ontario, Canada
[2]Kamloops Christian School, Kamloops, British Columbia, Canada

Chow et al. published a study in 2016 examining helmet use of adolescent boys at Crescent School, an independent all-boys day school, and reported a negative correlation. The aim of this study was to

---

* Correspondence: Ronald Chow BMSc(C), Bicycle Safety and Awareness Club, London, Ontario, Canada. Email: rchow48@uwo.ca.

determine the helmet use of adolescents at a co-educational independent school in the Province of British Columbia, Canada. A questionnaire was circulated to Grade 7 through 12 students at a high school. The questionnaire posed questions regarding bicycle-use on two occasions - the first instance was centred around bicycle-use as a means of transportation to arrive at the school, and the second focused on bicycle-use during recreational time. Seventeen students completed the questionnaire, with two remarking they are in Grade 7 and 8, six noting they are in Grade 9 and 10, and nine reporting they are in Grade 11 and 12. There seems to exist a negative correlation with respect to age and helmet use. There also seems to be a discrepancy between the proportion of students who are aware of the helmet legislation and those who regularly use a helmet; students knowingly choose not to use a helmet and not abide by the law. The reasons suggest an inherent inconvenience, and perhaps educational programs could focus on explaining how the extra effort of putting on a helmet has proven benefits in the event of an accident.

INTRODUCTION

Chow et al. (1) published a study in 2016 examining helmet use of adolescent boys at Crescent School, an independent all-boys day school. The authors reported a negative correlation - as age increases, the proportion of individuals who wear a helmet regularly decreases. 96% of students who were in Grade 7 and 8 used a helmet regularly, while only 59% of those in Grade 11 and 12 similarly used a helmet regularly.

A meta-analysis by Chow (2) revealed that other studies (3-8) have looked into this trend among adolescents. These studies looked into adolescents who attend schools with different student populations with respect to gender, geography and even school type (public school vs independent school). The original trend by Chow et al. (1) was confirmed, but there was variation between schools. The aim of this study was to determine the helmet use of adolescents at a high school in the Province of British Columbia, Canada.

OUR RESEARCH

A questionnaire was circulated to Grade 7 through 12 students at a high school in the Province of British Columbia, Canada. The objectives and analysis of this study are similar to those carried out by Chow et al. (1). The primary objectives of the survey were to determine (1) the percentage of cyclists at the school and (2) among those cyclists, the percentage who frequently wear a helmet. The questionnaire posed questions regarding bicycle-use on two occasions - the first instance was centred around bicycle-use as a means of transportation to arrive at the school, and the second focused on bicycle-use during recreational time. The secondary objective of the questionnaire was to determine the reasoning or motive of those who do not wear helmets, and subsequently gauge the students' knowledge on legislation around helmet-use. The questionnaire was anonymous, and students were strongly encouraged to complete the survey (9).

The data was analyzed by subgroups, based on the grade of participants - Grade 7 and 8, Grade 9 and 10, Grade 11 and 12. For questions pertaining to frequency of commute and frequency of helmet use, results were collapsed to yield two responses - "Always/Often" and "Rarely/On Occasion/Sometimes." The duration of the commute to school was also divided into two responses - "Under 20 minutes" and "Over 20 minutes." Fisher-exact test was used to examine the difference in proportions for multiple-choice results. Descriptive statistics were used for the short-answer question inquiring about helmet use. All analyses were performed using the Statistical Analysis Software (SAS Version 9.4 for Windows) (9).

FINDINGS

Seventeen students completed the questionnaire, with two remarking they are in Grade 7 and 8, six noting they are in Grade 9 and 10, and nine reporting they are in Grade 11 and 12. There was a smaller handful of older students who bike to school ($p = 0.0027$), with only 22% of Grade 11 and 12 students noting that they cycle to school while 100% of the younger grade students similarly reported so. 100% of the oldest cohort had short commutes, while 50% and 83% of the younger and middle age, respectively, similarly had short commutes ($p = 0.6667$). The three age groups, from youngest to oldest, had 100%, 83% and 50% of cyclists not commuting to school regularly ($p = 0.6667$). All cyclists noted that they regularly wear their helmets ($p = 0.9999$), and that they are aware a legislation about helmet use exists ($p = 0.9999$) (see Table 1).

As with the proportion of students who identify themselves as student cyclists, the older age group registered a smaller proportion who claimed they cycle during their recreational time ($p = 0.7731$); 67% as opposed to 100%. The majority of students use their helmet regularly during their recreational time ($p = 0.9999$), although 83% of the older group and 100% of the younger group regularly use a helmet. All students are aware of the legislation around helmet use ($p = 0.9999$) (see Table 2).

No reasons were provided for why student cyclists do not use a helmet when biking to school. Four reasons were provided by recreational cyclists - two by those in Grades 9 and 10, two by those in Grades 11 and 12 students. The two reasons provided by the younger group were split evenly across their desire not to carry their helmet around (50%) and their belief that they did not need one due to their short riding distance (50%). One (50%) Grade 11 and 12 student regarded that they cannot find their helmet and hence do not wear one, and another (50%) noted that they are normally in a rush (see Table 3).

Table 1. Demographics of cyclists to school

	Grades 7 & 8	Grades 9 & 10	Grades 11 & 12	*p*-value
Cyclist/Non-Cyclist				0.0027
Cyclist	2 (100%)	6 (100%)	2 (22%)	
Non-Cyclist	0 (0%)	0 (0%)	7 (78%)	
Duration				0.6667
Under 20 min	1 (50%)	5 (83%)	2 (100%)	
Over 20 min	1 (50%)	1 (17%)	0 (0%)	
Frequency of commute				0.6667
Always/Often	0 (0%)	1 (17%)	1 (50%)	
Rarely/On Occasion/Sometimes	2 (100%)	5 (83%)	1 (50%)	
Frequency of helmet use				0.9999
Always/Often	2 (100%)	6 (100%)	2 (100%)	
Rarely/On Occasion/Sometimes	0 (0%)	0 (0%)	0 (0%)	
Legislation about helmet use				0.9999
True	2 (100%)	6 (100%)	2 (100%)	
False	0 (0%)	0 (0%)	0 (0%)	

Table 2. Demographics of recreational cyclists

	Grades 7 & 8	Grades 9 & 10	Grades 11 & 12	*p*-value
Cyclist/Non-Cyclist				0.7731
Cyclist	2 (100%)	5 (83%)	6 (67%)	
Non-Cyclist	0 (0%)	1 (17%)	3 (33%)	
Frequency of helmet use				0.9999
Always/Often	2 (100%)	4 (80%)	5 (83%)	
Rarely/On Occasion/Sometimes	0 (0%)	1 (20%)	1 (17%)	
Legislation about helmet use				0.9999
True	2 (100%)	5 (100%)	6 (100%)	
False	0 (0%)	0 (0%)	0 (0%)	

Table 3. Reasons for not wearing a helmet - recreational cycling

Reasons	Grades 7 & 8	Grades 9 & 10	Grades 11 & 12
Do not like carrying it around	0 (0%)	1 (50%)	0 (0%)
Cannot find it	0 (0%)	0 (0%)	1 (50%)
In a rush	0 (0%)	0 (0%)	1 (50%)
Short distance	0 (0%)	1 (50%)	0 (0%)

DISCUSSION

The sample size of this study was very small, but the surveyed population in this study had a higher proportion of students who use a bicycle. Hence, even with the smaller sample population, the study still revealed some important results.

There were fewer older students who commute via bike to school than younger students, and those who do only commute a short distance. This may be a result of older students having other methods of commuting available to them, for example driving. Driving would be more prevalent among the older age group and would hence reduce the proportion of students who bike to school, particularly those who have a long commute time via a bicycle.

Among the population of recreational cyclists, there exists a discrepancy between the proportion of students who are aware of the helmet legislation and those who regularly use a helmet. In the younger cohort, such a discrepancy does not exist, as 100% of students both are aware of the law and regularly use a helmet. However, students in Grades 9 through 12 seem to be aware of the legislation yet choose not to regularly use a helmet. The reasons suggest an inherent inconvenience, and perhaps educational programs could focus on explaining how the extra effort of putting on a helmet has proven benefits in the event of an accident. The highest helmet wearing rate by the younger cohorts could also be a result of greater parental influence on decisions for younger individuals, hence helmet use increasing in prevalence as a result of the parental environment.

This study has its limitations. The sample size was very small and hence did not lead to high statistical power. Statistical trends could not be found, but quantitative trends can be suggested. Also, there exists the possibility of a response bias and a sampling bias as a result of the nature of the survey methods.

In conclusion, there seems to exist a negative correlation with respect to age and helmet use. There also seems to be a discrepancy between the proportion of students who are aware of the helmet legislation and those who regularly use a helmet; students knowingly choose not to use a helmet and not abide by the law. The reasons suggest an inherent inconvenience, and perhaps educational programs could teach that the extra effort to use a helmet has proven benefits in the event of an accident.

Acknowledgments

We would like to thank all of those who participated in the questionnaire.

References

[1] Chow R, Hollenberg D, Pintilie A, Midroni C, Cumner S. Helmet use of adolescent cyclists at Crescent School in Toronto, Canada. Int J Adolesc Med Health 2016, in press.

[2] Chow R. Bicycle and helmet use of young adults and adolescents: a meta-analysis. Int J Child Health Hum Dev 2018;11(1), in press.

[3] Borean M, Ho S, Hollenberg D, Anpalagan T, Rzepka A, Viehweger J, et al. Helmet use of adolescents in Markham, Canada. Int J Adolesc Med Health 2017, in press.

[4] Anpalagan T, Borean M, Chen L, Viehweger J, Hollenberg D, Rzepka A, et al. Helmet use of adolescents in Toronto, Canada. Int J Child Health Hum Dev 2018;11(1), in press.
[5] Borean M, Trasente V, Rzepka A, Viggiani D, Viotto D, Hollenberg D, et al. Helmet use of adolescents at De La Salle Oaklands in Toronto, Canada. Int J Child Health Hum Dev 2018;11(1), in press.
[6] Chow R, Borean M, Hollenberg D, Viehweger J, Young K, Southward N. Helmet use of adolescents at Ashbury College in Ottawa, Canada. Int J Child Health Hum Dev 2019, in press.
[7] Chow R, Borean M, Hollenberg D, Viehweger J, Hesse J. Helmet use of adolescents at Aberdeen Hall in Kelowna, Canada. Int J Child Health Hum Dev 2019, in press.
[8] Chow R, Borean M, Hollenberg D, Viehweger J, Alexander B, Gladstone J. Helmet use of adolescents at Linden School in Toronto, Canada. Int J Child Health Hum Dev 2019, in press.
[9] Chow R. Bicycle and helmet use: the survey instrument. Int J Child Health Hum Dev 2019, in press.

SECTION FOUR:
UNITED STATES OF AMERICA

In: Bicycles
Editors: Ronald Chow et al.

ISBN: 978-1-53612-458-3
© 2017 Nova Science Publishers, Inc.

Chapter 10

HELMET USE OF ADOLESCENTS AT AVON OLD FARMS SCHOOL IN AVON, UNITED STATES

Ronald Chow[*], *BMSc(C)*,
Jaclyn Viehweger, BMSc(C),
Michael Borean, BMSc(C)
and Drew Hollenberg, BMSc(C)
Bicycle Safety and Awareness Club, London, Ontario, Canada

The aim of this chapter was to investigate bicycle and helmet use of adolescents in Avon, CT, United States. A survey was circulated to Grade 9 through 12 students at Avon Old Farms School, an independent all-boys boarding school in Avon, CT, USA. The primary objectives of the survey were to determine 1) the percentage of cyclists at the school and 2) the percentage of cyclists who wear a helmet. The secondary objective of the questionnaire was to determine the reasoning or motive of those who do not wear helmets, and subsequently gauge the students'

---

[*] Correspondence: Ronald Chow BMSc(C), Bicycle Safety and Awareness Club, London, Ontario, Canada. Email: rchow48@uwo.ca.

knowledge on legislation around helmet-use. A total of 112 students completed the survey; 49 were in Grades 9 or 10, and 63 were in Grades 11 or 12. This is the first study to examine helmet use of adolescents in the United States and also amongst students in an all-boys independent boarding school. There seems to exist deviation in the results from prior studies, with lower proportion of students regularly using a helmet and aware of a helmet legislation. This may be a result of the safe environment established by the school and hence its students (who also reside at the school) do not feel that cycling could be a dangerous endeavour requiring a helmet on school premises. The negative correlation noted in literature is still observed, even with the noticeably different rates. Education programs can be established to increase the awareness of both the legislation and also the safety benefits offered by helmets.

INTRODUCTION

Many studies (1-8) have been conducted at Canadian independent schools to look into the helmet use of adolescents at various ages. The studies reported an inverse relationship between age and helmet use.

Chow et al. (1) noted that the proportion of adolescents who frequently wear a helmet fell from 96% to 59% at an independent all-boys day school in Toronto, Canada. Borean et al. (2) noted a similar decline from 88% to 58% at an independent co-ed day school also in Toronto, Canada. Studies conducted in other regions of Canada, such as British Columbia (6, 8) also reported a negative correlation.

Although a similar trend was observed across published studies, as reported in a meta-analysis (9), there also existed variation between studies. The aim of this study was to investigate bicycle and helmet use of adolescents in Avon, CT, USA.

OUR RESEARCH

A survey was circulated to Grade 9 through 12 students at Avon Old Farms School, an independent all-boys boarding school in Avon, CT, USA. The primary objectives of the survey were to determine 1) the percentage of cyclists at the school and 2) the percentage of cyclists who wear a helmet. The questionnaire posed questions regarding bicycle-use in two main instances - the first instance was centred around bicycle-use as a means of transportation to arrive at the school, and the second focused on bicycle-use during recreational time. The secondary objective of the questionnaire was to determine the reasoning or motive of those who do not wear helmets, and subsequently gauge the students' knowledge on legislation around helmet-use. The questionnaire was anonymous, and students were strongly encouraged to complete the survey (10).

The results of the questionnaire were examined by cohorts of grades - Grade 9 and 10, Grade 11 and 12. For questions pertaining to frequency of commute and frequency of helmet use, results were collapsed to yield two responses - "Always/Often" and "Rarely/On Occasion/Sometimes". The duration of the commute to school was also divided into two responses - "Under 20 minutes" and "Over 20 minutes." Fisher-exact test was used to examine the difference in proportions for multiple-choice results. Descriptive statistics were used for the short-answer question inquiring about helmet use. All analyses were performed using the Statistical Analysis Software (SAS Version 9.4 for Windows) (10).

FINDINGS

A total of 112 students completed the survey; 49 were in Grades 9 or 10, and 63 were in Grades 11 or 12. There seems to be a trend that a higher proportion of older students cycle to school or on school property (p = 0.1309); 32% of Grades 11 and 12 students identify as a cyclist as opposed to 18% of Grades 9 and 10 students. The majority of commutes are very short in duration (p = 0.6328), with 89% and 75% of the younger and older cohort, respectively, noting that their commute duration is under 20 minutes. There was virtually no difference between the two groups with respect to how often students commute via bike (p = 0.9999) - 95% of Grades 9 and 10 and 100% of Grades 11 and 12 students do not regularly bike. Only 33% and 35% of the groups, respectively, regularly use a helmet when biking (p = 0.9999). In those same two groups, 44% and 60% of students are aware that there exists a legislation mandating helmet use in Connecticut (p = 0.6882) (see Table 1).

Table 1. Demographics of cyclists to school

	Grades 9 & 10	Grades 11 & 12	p-value
Cyclist/Non-Cyclist			0.1309
Cyclist	9 (18%)	20 (32%)	
Non-Cyclist	40 (82%)	43 (68%)	
Duration			0.6328
Under 20 min	8 (89%)	15 (75%)	
Over 20 min	1 (11%)	5 (25%)	
Frequency of commute			0.9999
Always/Often	0 (0%)	1 (5%)	
Rarely/On Occasion/Sometimes	9 (100%)	19 (95%)	
Frequency of helmet use			0.9999
Always/Often	3 (33%)	7 (35%)	
Rarely/On Occasion/Sometimes	6 (67%)	13 (65%)	
Legislation about helmet use			0.6882
True	4 (44%)	12 (60%)	
False	5 (56%)	8 (40%)	

Table 2. Demographics of recreational cyclists

	Grades 9 & 10	Grades 11 & 12	*p*-value
Cyclist/Non-Cyclist			0.6721
Cyclist	37 (76%)	45 (71%)	
Non-Cyclist	12 (25%)	18 (29%)	
Frequency of helmet use			0.2239
Always/Often	13 (35%)	10 (22%)	
Rarely/On Occasion/Sometimes	24 (65%)	35 (78%)	
Legislation about helmet use			0.2662
True	18 (49%)	28 (62%)	
False	19 (51%)	17 (38%)	

Table 3. Reasons for not wearing a helmet - school commute

Reasons	Grades 9 & 10	Grades 11 & 12
Can't find it	2 (50%)	0 (0%)
Inconvenient/Nowhere to put it	1 (25%)	1 (9%)
Looks stupid	1 (25%)	0 (0%)
Don't need one/Won't help me if I get hit	0 (0%)	8 (73%)
Other*:	0 (0%)	2 (18%)

* Other: Helmets are uncomfortable.

Table 4. Reasons for not wearing a helmet - recreational cycling

Reasons	Grades 9 & 10	Grades 11 & 12
Helmets are uncomfortable	5 (24%)	7 (28%)
Don't need one/Short safe trip	9 (43%)	15 (60%)
Looks stupid	2 (10%)	1 (4%)
Inconvenient	2 (10%)	2 (8%)
Can't find it	2 (10%)	0 (0%)
Other*	1 (5%)	0 (0%)

* Other: Do not have a helmet.

Approximately three-quarters of students reported that they ride a bicycle during their recreational time (p = 0.6721), with 76% of Grade 9 and 10, 71% of Grade 11 and 12 remarking so. There seems to be an indication that older students do not use their helmets as regularly (p = 0.2239), with 22% regularly using a helmet as opposed to 35%. The older group may be more informed about the existing legislation around helmet use (p = 0.2662) - 62% noted there exists a legislation among Grade 11 and 12 students, while a lower 49% of Grade 9 and 12 students reported that there exists such a legislation (see Table 2).

4 and 11 reasons were provided by students by the older and younger age cohort, respectively, as to why they do not use a helmet during their school commute. The most common reason (50%) by the younger group was that they cannot find their helmet; other reasons included inconvenience and cosmetic appearance (25% each). The older cohort most often cited (73%) that they do not need a helmet and that it would not help them in the event of a collision, while also noting the uncomfortable (18%) and inconvenient (9%) nature of helmets (see Table 3).

Among students who identified themselves as a recreational cyclist, 21 reasons were provided by Grades 9 and 10 students and 25 responses were noted from Grades 11 and 12 students. Grades 9 and 10 students most commonly cited that they bike short distances (43%), followed by noting the uncomfortable nature (24%) as a deterrent to using a helmet. Other reasons included cosmetic reasons (10%), inconvenience (10%), inability to find their helmet (10%), and that they do not have one (5%). The older group similarly mainly cited that they do not need a helmet due to the short distance (60%), with other reasons being uncomfort (28%), inconvenience (8%) and physical appearances (4%) (see Table 4).

DISCUSSION

This is the first study to examine helmet use of adolescents in the United States of America, and also the first to look at helmet use of adolescents at an all-boys independent boarding school. The results, when compared with those previously documented in literature, suggests that there does exist variation by region.

There exists a very low percentage of students who regularly cycle to school. This is a result of the nature of the school environment. Boarding school allows for students to live in close proximity to the school and hence would not necessitate the use of a bicycle to reduce commute times.

The proportion of students who regularly use a helmet in this cohort is much lower than those reported in prior studies. This may be a result of a different childhood environment. It may also be a direct consequence of the lower awareness of legislation regarding helmets as opposed to other regions. However, it could also be a result of the safe environment established by the school and hence its students (who also reside at the school) do not feel that cycling could be a dangerous endeavour requiring a helmet on school premises. Nevertheless, education programs can be established to increase the awareness of both the legislation and also the safety benefits offered by helmets.

Even though there exists deviance from prior studies, the negative correlation between age and helmet use still seems to persist. The change, although not statistical significant, is quantitatively remarkable (22% in the older group, from 35% in the younger group) and may have been noted as a substantial difference if a larger sample population had been accrued.

This study was not without limitations. As with any survey, there exists the possibility of a response bias. Additionally, as the survey was circulated around to students via media outlets (i.e., school portals, email system) and advertised as optional, there also exists the potential for a sampling bias. These biases were hopefully minimized by accruing a substantial sample size, but p-values yielded should still be interpreted with caution.

In conclusion, this is the first study to examine helmet use of adolescents in the United States and also amongst students in an all-boys independent boarding school. There seems to exist deviation in the results from prior studies, with lower proportion of students regularly using a helmet and aware of a helmet legislation. This may be a result of the safe environment established by the school and hence its students (who also reside at the school) do not feel that cycling could be a dangerous endeavour requiring a helmet on school premises. The negative correlation noted in literature is still observed, even with the noticeably different rates. Education programs can be established to increase the awareness of both the legislation and also the safety benefits offered by helmets.

Acknowledgments

We would like to thank all of those who participated in the questionnaire.

References

[1] Chow R, Hollenberg D, Pintilie A, Midroni C, Cumner S. Helmet use of adolescent cyclists at Crescent School in Toronto, Canada. Int J Adolesc Med Health 2016, in press.

[2] Borean M, Ho S, Hollenberg D, Anpalagan T, Rzepka A, Viehweger J, et al. Helmet use of adolescents in Markham, Canada. Int J Adolesc Med Health 2017, in press.

[3] Anpalagan T, Borean M, Chen L, Viehweger J, Hollenberg D, Rzepka A, et al. Helmet use of adolescents in Toronto, Canada. Int J Child Health Hum Dev 2018;11(1), in press.

[4] Borean M, Trasente V, Rzepka A, Viggiani D, Viotto D, Hollenberg D, et al. Helmet use of adolescents at De La Salle Oaklands in Toronto, Canada. Int J Child Health Hum Dev 2018;11(1), in press.

[5] Chow R, Borean M, Hollenberg D, Viehweger J, Young K, Southward N. Helmet use of adolescents at Ashbury College in Ottawa, Canada. Int J Child Health Hum Dev 2019, in press.

[6] Chow R, Borean M, Hollenberg D, Viehweger J, Hesse J. Helmet use of adolescents at Aberdeen Hall in Kelowna, Canada. Int J Child Health Hum Dev 2019, in press.

[7] Chow R, Borean M, Hollenberg D, Viehweger J, Alexander B, Gladstone J. Helmet use of adolescents at Linden School in Toronto, Canada. Int J Child Health Hum Dev 2019, in press.

[8] Viehweger J, Borean M, Hollenberg D, Cuzzetto S, Chow R. Helmet use of adolescents at Kamloops Christian School in Kamloops, Canada. Int J Child Health Hum Dev 2019, in press.

[9] Chow R. Bicycle and helmet use of young adults and adolescents: a meta-analysis. Int J Child Health Hum Dev 2018;11(1), in press.

[10] Chow R. Bicycle and helmet use: the survey instrument. Int J Child Health Hum Dev 2019, in press.

Section five: Overall

In: Bicycles
Editors: Ronald Chow et al.

ISBN: 978-1-53612-458-3
© 2017 Nova Science Publishers, Inc.

Chapter 11

BICYCLE AND HELMET USE OF ADOLESCENTS: A META-ANALYSIS

Ronald Chow[*], BMSc(C),
Michael Borean, BMSc(C),
Drew Hollenberg, BMSc(C),
Jaclyn Viehweger, BMSc(C),
Tharani Anpalagan, BMSc(C)
and Anna Rzepka, BMSc(C)
Bicycle Safety and Awareness Club, London, Ontario, Canada

A prior meta-analysis suggested that there seems to exist a negative correlation between age and helmet use among adolescents. Since the meta-analysis, multiple new literature has been published that have also looked into helmet use of adolescents. The aim of this meta-analysis is to update the prior meta-analysis and include the data from new studies. A literature search was conducted in many databases, such as Ovid

---

[*] Correspondence: Ronald Chow BMSc(C), Bicycle Safety and Awareness Club, London, Ontario, Canada. Email: rchow48@uwo.ca.

MEDLINE and OLDMEDLINE, Embase Classic and Embase, PsycINFO. Relevant studies were screened to determine whether it reported bicycle and helmet use in adolescent. Data from the prior meta-analysis was also included. The extracted endpoints were: bicycle use when commuting to school, duration of school commute, frequency of school commute, frequency of helmet use during school commute, knowledge of legislation/safety, bicycle use during recreational time, and frequency of helmet use during recreational time. A total of 12 studies were included in this meta-analysis, of which fifteen datasets were included. This meta-analysis with a much larger sample population verifies the negative correlation that was previously noted in an earlier meta-analysis. Among students who cycle to school, the frequency of helmet use fell from 82% to 50%, while it fell from 82% to 52% among recreational cyclists.

INTRODUCTION

Helmets have been documented to be effective in reducing the number of head injuries after head trauma from bicycle accidents (1). However, studies have suggested that the adoption of helmet use among cyclists is not high – many cyclists do not regularly use a helmet.

A meta-analysis was previously published (2), and documented helmet use of young adults (3-15) adolescents. In the young adult population, there exists a positive correlation between age and helmet use; as young adults grow older, the proportion of cyclists who were a helmet regularly increases.

The meta-analysis also included some studies that documented helmet use of adolescents. Chow et al. conducted a study at an independent single-sex school in Toronto, Canada, and observed that among adolescent boys, helmet use fell from 96% to 59% (16). Borean et al. also noted a similar decline from 88% to 58% at a public co-educational school in Markham (Greater Toronto Area), Canada (17).

Since the meta-analysis, multiple new literature has been published that have also looked into helmet use of adolescents (18-20). The aim of this meta-analysis is to update the prior meta-analysis and include the data from new studies.

LITERATURE SEARCH

A literature search was conducted in many databases, such as Ovid MEDLINE and OLDMEDLINE, Embase Classic and Embase, PsycINFO. Relevant studies were screened to determine whether it reported bicycle and helmet use in adolescent. Data from the prior meta-analysis was also included.

The extracted endpoints were: bicycle use when commuting to school, duration of school commute, frequency of school commute, frequency of helmet use during school commute, knowledge of legislation/safety, bicycle use during recreational time, and frequency of helmet use during recreational time. These endpoints were compiled into a table and summed to produce a weighted average for each endpoint among independent schools, public schools and schools outside of North America. The endpoints were produced for six age cohorts – three cohorts of adolescents (Grade 7-8 students, Grade 9-10 students, Grade 11-12 students) and three cohorts of young adults (aged 19 years and below, between 20 and 22 years old, and 23 years old and above).

STUDIES FOUND

A total of 12 studies were included in this meta-analysis (16-27), of which fifteen datasets were included. Ten sets documented helmet use of Grade 7 through 12 students at independent schools, one disclosed helmet use of Grade 7 to 8 students at independent schools and another of Grade 9 to 12 at another independent school, two reported on helmet use of Grade 9 to 12 at public schools, and another of a high school outside of North America.

Table 1. Bicycle and helmet use of (grade 7-8) adolescents, to school

Study	School Cyclist Cyclist	School Cyclist Non-Cyclist	Duration Under 20 Min	Duration Over 20 Min	Frequency of Commute Always/Often	Frequency of Commute Rarely/On Occasion/Sometimes	Frequency of Helmet Use Always/Often	Frequency of Helmet Use Rarely/On Occasion/Sometimes	Educated of Legislation Educated	Educated of Legislation Uneducated
Chow et al. 2016 (16)	46 (46%)	55 (54%)	41 (89%)	5 (12%)	9 (20%)	37 (80%)	44 (96%)	2 (4%)	41 (89%)	5 (11%)
Borean et al. 2018 (18)	5 (14%)	32 (85%)	4 (80%)	1 (20%)	4 (80%)	1 (20%)	4 (80%)	1 (20%)	4 (80%)	1 (20%)
Chow et al. (2)	2 (8%)	22 (92%)	2 (100%)	0 (0%)	0 (0%)	2 (100%)	1 (50%)	1 (50%)	1 (50%)	1 (50%)
Chow et al. (19)	29 (35%)	53 (65%)	26 (90%)	3 (10%)	4 (14%)	25 (86%)	22 (76%)	7 (24%)	23 (79%)	6 (21%)
Chow et al. (20)	0 (0%)	9 (100%)	0 (0%)	0 (0%)	0 (0%)	0 (0%)	0 (0%)	0 (0%)	0 (0%)	0 (0%)
Chow et al. (21)	2 (20%)	8 (80%)	0 (0%)	2 (100%)	0 (0%)	2 (100%)	2 (100%)	0 (0%)	2 (100%)	0 (0%)
Viehweger et al. (22)	2 (100%)	0 (0%)	1 (50%)	1 (50%)	0 (0%)	2 (100%)	2 (100%)	0 (0%)	2 (100%)	0 (0%)
Chow et al. (23)	11 (19%)	47 (81%)	7 (64%)	4 (36%)	1 (9%)	10 (91%)	5 (45%)	6 (56%)	9 (82%)	2 (18%)
Chow et al. (24)	6 (23%)	20 (77%)	3 (50%)	3 (50%)	1 (17%)	5 (83%)	5 (83%)	1 (17%)	3 (50%)	3 (50%)
Chow et al. (25)	16 (30%)	37 (70%)	15 (94%)	1 (6%)	4 (25%)	12 (75%)	12 (75%)	4 (25%)	15 (94%)	1 (6%)
Independent School	*119 (30%)*	*283 (70%)*	*99 (83%)*	*20 (17%)*	*23 (19%)*	*96 (81%)*	*97 (82%)*	*22 (19%)*	*100 (84%)*	*19 (16%)*
Total	119 (30%)	283 (70%)	99 (83%)	20 (17%)	23 (19%)	96 (81%)	97 (82%)	22 (19%)	100 (84%)	19 (16%)

Table 2. Bicycle and helmet use of (grade 7-8) adolescents, during recreational time

Study	Recreational Cyclist		Frequency of Helmet Use			Educated of Legislation	
	Cyclist	Non-Cyclist	Always/Often	Rarely/On Occasion/Sometimes		Educated	Uneducated
Chow et al. 2016 (16)	93 (92%)	8 (8%)	82 (88%)	11 (12%)		85 (91%)	8 (9%)
Borean et al. 2018 (18)	27 (73%)	10 (27%)	20 (74%)	7 (26%)		17 (63%)	10 (37%)
Chow et al. (2)	19 (79%)	5 (21%)	16 (84%)	3 (16%)		18 (95%)	1 (5%)
Chow et al. (19)	71 (87%)	11 (13%)	58 (82%)	13 (18%)		59 (83%)	12 (17%)
Chow et al. (20)	8 (89%)	1 (11%)	7 (88%)	1 (12%)		5 (62%)	3 (38%)
Chow et al. (21)	9 (90%)	1 (10%)	9 (100%)	0 (0%)		8 (89%)	1 (11%)
Viehweger et al. (22)	2 (100%)	0 (0%)	2 (100%)	0 (0%)		2 (100%)	0 (0%)
Chow et al. (23)	48 (83%)	10 (17%)	32 (67%)	16 (33%)		43 (90%)	5 (10%)
Chow et al. (24)	24 (92%)	2 (8%)	19 (79%)	5 (21%)		15 (63%)	9 (38%)
Chow et al. (25)	51 (96%)	2 (4%)	45 (88%)	6 (12%)		45 (88%)	6 (12%)
Independent School	*352 (88%)*	*50 (12%)*	*290 (82%)*	*62 (18%)*		*297 (84%)*	*55 (16%)*
Total	352 (88%)	50 (12%)	290 (82%)	62 (18%)		297 (84%)	55 (16%)

Table 3. Bicycle and helmet use of (grade 9-10) adolescents, to school

Study	School Cyclist Cyclist	School Cyclist Non-Cyclist	Duration Under 20 Min	Duration Over 20 Min	Frequency of Commute Always/Often	Frequency of Commute Rarely/On Occasion/Sometimes	Frequency of Helmet Use Always/Often	Frequency of Helmet Use Rarely/On Occasion/Sometimes	Educated of Legislation Educated	Educated of Legislation Uneducated
Chow et al. 2016 (16)	45 (46%)	53 (54%)	39 (87%)	6 (13%)	6 (13%)	39 (87%)	34 (76%)	11 (24%)	44 (98%)	1 (2%)
Borean et al. 2018 (18)	8 (11%)	63 (89%)	7 (88%)	1 (13%)	2 (25%)	6 (75%)	5 (63%)	3 (38%)	7 (88%)	1 (13%)
Chow et al. (19)	4 (15%)	23 (85%)	3 (75%)	1 (25%)	1 (25%)	3 (75%)	1 (25%)	3 (75%)	4 (100%)	0 (0%)
Chow et al. (20)	1 (7%)	13 (93%)	1 (100%)	0 (0%)	0 (0%)	1 (100%)	0 (0%)	1 (100%)	1 (100%)	0 (0%)
Chow et al. (21)	1 (14%)	6 (86%)	0 (0%)	1 (100%)	0 (0%)	1 (100%)	1 (100%)	0 (0%)	1 (100%)	0 (0%)
Viehweger et al. (22)	6 (100%)	0 (0%)	5 (83%)	1 (17%)	1 (17%)	5 (83%)	6 (100%)	0 (0%)	6 (100%)	0 (0%)
Chow et al. (26)	9 (18%)	40 (82%)	8 (89%)	1 (11%)	0 (0%)	9 (100%)	3 (33%)	6 (67%)	4 (44%)	5 (56%)
Chow et al. (23)	13 (15%)	73 (85%)	8 (62%)	5 (38%)	3 (23%)	10 (77%)	7 (54%)	6 (46%)	9 (69%)	4 (31%)
Chow et al. (24)	7 (22%)	25 (78%)	2 (29%)	5 (71%)	0 (0%)	7 (100%)	3 (43%)	4 (57%)	2 (29%)	5 (71%)
Chow et al. (25)	9 (25%)	27 (75%)	5 (56%)	4 (44%)	0 (0%)	9 (100%)	8 (89%)	1 (11%)	9 (100%)	0 (0%)
Independent School	103	323	78	25	13	90	68	35	87	16

Study	School Cyclist		Duration		Frequency of Commute		Frequency of Helmet Use		Educated of Legislation	
	Cyclist	Non-Cyclist	Under 20 Min	Over 20 Min	Always/Often	Rarely/On Occasion/Sometimes	Always/Often	Rarely/On Occasion/Sometimes	Educated	Uneducated
	(24%)	*(76%)*	*(76%)*	*(24%)*	*(13%)*	*(87%)*	*(66%)*	*(34%)*	*(84%)*	*(16%)*
Borean et al. 2017 (17)	7 *(26%)*	20 *(74%)*	7 *(100%)*	0 *(0%)*	0 *(0%)*	7 *(100%)*	1 *(14%)*	6 *(86%)*	6 *(86%)*	1 *(14%)*
Anpalagan et al. 2018 (27)	6 *(13%)*	41 *(87%)*	4 *(67%)*	2 *(33%)*	0 *(0%)*	6 *(100%)*	5 *(83%)*	1 *(17%)*	5 *(83%)*	1 *(17%)*
Public School	13 *(18%)*	61 *(82%)*	11 *(85%)*	2 *(15%)*	0 *(0%)*	13 *(100%)*	6 *(46%)*	7 *(54%)*	11 *(85%)*	2 *(15%)*
Total	116 *(23%)*	384 *(77%)*	89 *(77%)*	27 *(23%)*	13 *(11%)*	103 *(89%)*	74 *(64%)*	42 *(36%)*	98 *(85%)*	18 *(16%)*

Table 4. Bicycle and helmet use of (grade 9-10) adolescents, during recreational time

Study	Recreational Cyclist		Frequency of Helmet Use		Educated of Legislation	
	Cyclist	Non-Cyclist	Always/Often	Rarely/On Occasion/Sometimes	Educated	Uneducated
Chow et al. 2016 (16)	88 *(89%)*	11 *(11%)*	53 *(60%)*	35 *(40%)*	80 *(91%)*	8 *(9%)*
Borean et al. 2018 (18)	58 *(82%)*	13 *(18%)*	38 *(66%)*	20 *(34%)*	45 *(78%)*	13 *(22%)*
Chow et al. (19)	25 *(93%)*	2 *(7%)*	12 *(48%)*	13 *(52%)*	22 *(88%)*	3 *(12%)*
Chow et al. (20)	13 *(93%)*	1 *(7%)*	7 *(54%)*	6 *(46%)*	11 *(85%)*	2 *(15%)*

Table 4. (Continued)

Study	Recreational Cyclist		Frequency of Helmet Use			Educated of Legislation	
	Cyclist	Non-Cyclist	Always/Often	Rarely/On Occasion/Sometimes		Educated	Uneducated
Chow et al. (21)	6 (86%)	1 (14%)	5 (83%)	1 (17%)		5 (83%)	1 (17%)
Viehweger et al. (22)	5 (83%)	1 (17%)	4 (80%)	1 (20%)		5 (100%)	0 (0%)
Chow et al. (26)	37 (76%)	12 (25%)	13 (35%)	24 (65%)		18 (49%)	19 (51%)
Chow et al. (23)	68 (79%)	18 (21%)	46 (68%)	22 (32%)		57 (84%)	11 (16%)
Chow et al. (24)	24 (75%)	8 (25%)	17 (71%)	7 (29%)		19 (79%)	5 (21%)
Chow et al. (25)	25 (69%)	11 (31%)	19 (76%)	6 (24%)		22 (88%)	3 (12%)
Independent School	*349 (82%)*	*78 (18%)*	*214 (61%)*	*135 (39%)*		*284 (81%)*	*65 (19%)*
Borean et al. 2017 (17)	17 (63%)	10 (37%)	7 (41%)	10 (59%)		16 (94%)	1 (6%)
Anpalagan et al. 2018 (27)	38 (81%)	9 (19%)	23 (61%)	15 (39%)		32 (84%)	6 (16%)
Public School	*55 (74%)*	*19 (26%)*	*30 (55%)*	*25 (45%)*		*48 (87%)*	*7 (13%)*
Total	404 (81%)	97 (19%)	244 (60%)	160 (40%)		332 (82%)	72 (18%)

Table 5. Bicycle and helmet use of (grade 11-12) adolescents, to school

Study	School Cyclist Cyclist	School Cyclist Non-Cyclist	Duration Under 20 Min	Duration Over 20 Min	Frequency of Commute Always/Often	Frequency of Commute Rarely/On Occasion/Sometimes	Frequency of Helmet Use Always/Often	Frequency of Helmet Use Rarely/On Occasion/Sometimes	Educated of Legislation Educated	Educated of Legislation Uneducated
Chow et al. 2016 (16)	29 (51%)	28 (49%)	20 (69%)	9 (31%)	4 (14%)	25 (86%)	17 (59%)	12 (41%)	23 (79%)	6 (21%)
Borean et al. 2018 (18)	20 (16%)	106 (84%)	10 (50%)	10 (50%)	0 (0%)	20 (100%)	11 (55%)	9 (45%)	14 (70%)	6 (30%)
Chow et al. (19)	2 (7%)	26 (93%)	2 (100%)	0 (0%)	1 (50%)	1 (50%)	1 (50%)	1 (50%)	1 (50%)	1 (50%)
Chow et al. (20)	1 (9%)	10 (91%)	1 (100%)	0 (0%)	0 (0%)	1 (100%)	0 (0%)	1 (100%)	0 (0%)	1 (100%)
Chow et al. (21)	3 (33%)	6 (67%)	1 (33%)	2 (67%)	0 (0%)	3 (100%)	1 (33%)	2 (67%)	1 (33%)	2 (67%)
Viehweger et al. (22)	2 (22%)	7 (78%)	2 (100%)	0 (0%)	1 (50%)	1 (50%)	2 (100%)	0 (0%)	2 (100%)	0 (0%)
Chow et al. (26)	20 (32%)	43 (68%)	15 (75%)	5 (25%)	1 (5%)	19 (95%)	7 (35%)	13 (65%)	12 (60%)	8 (40%)
Chow et al. (23)	15 (18%)	67 (82%)	13 (87%)	2 (13%)	2 (13%)	13 (87%)	8 (53%)	7 (47%)	4 (27%)	11 (73%)
Chow et al. (24)	4 (21%)	15 (79%)	4 (100%)	0 (0%)	2 (50%)	2 (50%)	2 (50%)	2 (50%)	4 (100%)	0 (0%)
Chow et al. (25)	5 (16%)	27 (84%)	3 (60%)	2 (40%)	0 (0%)	5 (100%)	3 (60%)	2 (40%)	5 (100%)	0 (0%)

Table 5. (Continued)

Study	School Cyclist		Duration		Frequency of Commute		Frequency of Helmet Use		Educated of Legislation	
	Cyclist	Non-Cyclist	Under 20 Min	Over 20 Min	Always/Often	Rarely/On Occasion/Sometimes	Always/Often	Rarely/On Occasion/Sometimes	Educated	Uneducated
Independent School	101 (23%)	335 (77%)	71 (70%)	30 (30%)	11 (11%)	90 (89%)	52 (51%)	49 (49%)	66 (65%)	35 (35%)
Borean et al. 2017 (17)	27 (23%)	90 (77%)	20 (74%)	7 (26%)	4 (15%)	23 (85%)	8 (30%)	19 (70%)	24 (89%)	3 (11%)
Anpalagan et al. 2018 (27)	21 (27%)	58 (73%)	11 (52%)	10 (48%)	3 (14%)	18 (86%)	15 (71%)	6 (29%)	16 (76%)	5 (24%)
Public School	48 (24%)	148 (76%)	31 (65%)	17 (35%)	7 (15%)	41 (85%)	23 (48%)	25 (52%)	40 (83%)	8 (17%)
Chow et al. (2)	0 (0%)	12 (100%)	0 (0%)	0 (0%)	0 (0%)	0 (0%)	0 (0%)	0 (0%)	0 (0%)	0 (0%)
Outside of North America	0 (0%)	12 (100%)	0 (0%)	0 (0%)	0 (0%)	0 (0%)	0 (0%)	0 (0%)	0 (0%)	0 (0%)
Total	149 (23%)	495 (77%)	102 (68%)	47 (32%)	18 (12%)	131 (88%)	75 (50%)	74 (50%)	106 (71%)	43 (29%)

Grade 7-8 adolescents

Only independent school students were surveyed. 30% of students identified noted that they use a bicycle to commute to school. 83% have a commute duration of under 20 minutes, and 19% of students regularly commute. 82% regularly use a helmet when commuting. 84% of students are aware of bicycle helmet legislation (see Table 1).

88% identified themselves as recreational cyclists. While 82% of students regularly used a helmet when commuting, 84% were knowledgeable about the helmet legislation (see Table 2).

Grade 9-10 adolescents

24% of independent school students used a bike to commute to school. Of this cohort, 76% have a short commute, 13% regularly commute, 66% regularly use a helmet, and 84% were aware of helmet legislation (see Table 3).

Among public school students, 18% noted that they use a bicycle to commute to school. 85% of students reported that they have a short commute, with all of them noting that they do regularly commute. While 46% of students do not regularly use a helmet, 85% of these students were aware of helmet use legislation (see Table 3).

Overall, between independent and public school students, 23% identified themselves as cyclists who commute to school. 77% reported that their commute time is less than 20 minutes and only 11% regularly commuted using a bike. 64% noted that they regularly use a helmet when commuting. 85% of the students were aware of the bicycle helmet legislation (see Table 3).

82% of independent school students and 74% of public school students identified recreational cyclists, and regularly used a helmet at a frequency of 61% and 55%, respectively. 81% and 87% of recreational cyclists who attended independent and public schools, respectively, were aware of the helmet legislation. Overall, 81% of students cycle during their recreational time, 60% regularly use a helmet, and 82% were aware of the bicycle legislation (see Table 4).

Grade 11-12 adolescents

23% of students commuted to school – 24% for public school and 23% for independent school students. 65% of public school students, 71% of independent school students, and 68% overall, noted that their commute to school takes under 20 minutes via bike. 15%, 11% and 12% of those groups, respectively, noted that they regularly commute using a bike. 48% and 83% of the public school students used a helmet regularly and were aware of the helmet legislation, respectively. 51% and 65% were the metrics were independent school students; for students in general, it was 50% and 71% (see Table 5).

While 75% of independent school students used a bicycle during their recreational time, 68% of public school students and 33% of students outside of North America similarly reported so. 56%, 43% and 0% of the cohorts, respectively, regularly use a helmet when biking. 78%, 81% and 100% noted that they are aware of a bicycle helmet legislation. Overall, 72% of students use a bike during their recreational time, of which 52% regularly use a helmet and 79% are aware of the helmet legislation (see Table 6).

DISCUSSION

This meta-analysis includes twelve studies looking into helmet use of adolescents as opposed to three in a prior meta-analysis (2). The much larger sample size verifies the trend previously noted – there exists a negative correlation between age and helmet use. Among those who commute to school, the proportion of students who regularly use a helmet falls from 82% to 64% to 50%. For recreational cyclists, the percentage fell from 82% to 60% to 52%.

Table 6. Bicycle and helmet use of (grade 11-12) adolescents, during recreational time

Study	Recreational Cyclist		Frequency of Helmet Use		Educated of Legislation	
	Cyclist	Non-Cyclist	Always/Often	Rarely/On Occasion/Sometimes	Educated	Uneducated
Chow et al. 2016 (16)	45 (79%)	12 (21%)	26 (58%)	19 (42%)	37 (82%)	8 (18%)
Borean et al. 2018 (18)	104 (83%)	22 (17%)	57 (55%)	47 (45%)	82 (79%)	22 (21%)
Chow et al. (19)	20 (71%)	8 (29%)	14 (70%)	6 (30%)	16 (80%)	4 (20%)
Chow et al. (20)	9 (82%)	2 (18%)	8 (89%)	1 (11%)	7 (78%)	2 (22%)
Chow et al. (21)	5 (56%)	4 (44%)	2 (40%)	3 (60%)	1 (20%)	4 (80%)
Viehweger et al. (22)	6 (67%)	3 (33%)	5 (83%)	1 (17%)	6 (100%)	0 (0%)
Chow et al. (26)	45 (71%)	18 (29%)	10 (22%)	35 (78%)	28 (62%)	17 (38%)
Chow et al. (23)	55 (67%)	27 (33%)	38 (69%)	17 (31%)	46 (84%)	9 (16%)
Chow et al. (24)	13 (68%)	6 (32%)	10 (77%)	3 (23%)	10 (77%)	3 (23%)
Chow et al. (25)	25 (78%)	7 (22%)	13 (52%)	12 (48%)	21 (84%)	4 (16%)
Independent School	*327 (75%)*	*109 (25%)*	*183 (56%)*	*144 (44%)*	*254 (78%)*	*73 (22%)*
Borean et al. 2017 (17)	78 (67%)	39 (33%)	30 (38%)	48 (62%)	65 (83%)	13 (17%)
Anpalagan et al. 2018 (27)	56 (71%)	23 (29%)	28 (50%)	28 (50%)	44 (79%)	12 (21%)
Public School	*134 (68%)*	*62 (32%)*	*58 (43%)*	*76 (57%)*	*109 (81%)*	*25 (19%)*
Chow et al. (2)	4 (33%)	8 (66%)	0 (0%)	4 (100%)	4 (100%)	0 (0%)
Outside of North America	*4 (33%)*	*8 (66%)*	*0 (0%)*	*4 (100%)*	*4 (100%)*	*0 (0%)*
Total	465 (72%)	179 (28%)	241 (52%)	224 (48%)	367 (79%)	98 (21%)

Independent school students seem to use helmets more regularly than public school students. It is important to note, however, that only two studies have documented helmet use among the public school students and hence the findings may just be anomalies.

The percentage of students who regularly use a helmet is less than the proportion of students who are aware of the bicycle legislation. It hence seems that adolescents have a disregard for the bicycle helmet legislation, and prefer the convenience, comfort and appearance of not using a helmet.

This review was not without limitations. There was no statistical procedures conducted to determine whether the differences between age cohorts in this group was significant. A future study should look into repeating this analysis with statistical procedures.

In conclusion, this meta-analysis with a much larger sample population verifies the negative correlation that was previously noted in an earlier meta-analysis. Among students who cycle to school, the frequency of helmet use fell from 82% to 50%, while it fell from 82% to 52% among recreational cyclists.

ACKNOWLEDGMENTS

I would like to thank the Bicycle Safety and Awareness Club for all their work in the published primary research, and also for their work in collecting unpublished primary research data. I would like to thank Michael Borean, Drew Hollenberg, Tharani Anpalagan, Anna Rzepka and Jaclyn Viehweger in their support and assistance of the preparation of this manuscript.

REFERENCES

[1] Attewell RG, Glase K, McFadden M. Bicycle helmet efficacy: a meta-analysis. Accid Anal Prev 2001;33(3):345-52.

[2] Chow R. Bicycle and helmet use of young adults and adolescents: a meta-analysis. Int J Child Health Hum Dev 2018;11(1), in press.

[3] Chow R, Borean M, Hollenberg D, Ganguli N, Freedman Z, Kang R, et al. Helmet use of young adults in New York State, United States of America. Int J Child Health Hum Dev 2018;11(1), in press.

[4] Anpalagan T, Hollenberg D, Borean M, Rzepka A, Chow R. Helmet use of young adults in London, Canada. Int J Child Health Hum Dev 2018;11(1), in press.

[5] Anpalagan T, Panigrahi I, Borean M, Hollenberg D, Rzepka A, Viehweger J et al. Helmet use of young adults in Hamilton, Canada. Int J Child Health Hum Dev 2018;11(1), in press.

[6] Rzepka A, Borean M, Hollenberg D, Chan Z, Binns A, Weise E, et al. Helmet use of young adults in Guelph, Canada. Int J Child Health Hum Dev 2018;11(1), in press.

[7] Anpalagan T, Duarte N, Borean M, Anpalagan J, Camilleri R, Hollenberg D, et al. Helmet use of young adults in Waterloo, Canada. Int J Child Health Hum Dev 2018;11(1), in press.

[8] Chow R, Borean M, Hollenberg D, Ho C, Ng W, Guo W, et al. Helmet use of young adults in Toronto, Canada. Int J Child Health Hum Dev 2018;11(1), in press.

[9] Viehweger J, Borean M, Tang M, Hollenberg D, Anpalagan T, Rzepka A, et al. Helmet use of young adults in St. Catherines, Canada. Int J Child Health Hum Dev 2018;11(1), in press.

[10] Viehweger J, Borean M, Midroni L, Midroni C, Hollenberg D, Anpalagan T et al. Helmet use of young adults in Kingston, Canada. Int J Child Health Hum Dev 2018;11(1), in press.

[11] Chow R, Borean M, Hollenberg D, Song K, Liu J, Young T, et al. Helmet use of young adults in Montreal, Canada. Int J Child Health Hum Dev 2018;11(1), in press.

[12] Chow R, Rzepka A, Borean M, Parekh R, Hollenberg D, Anpalagan T, et al. Helmet use of young adults in Saskatoon, Canada. Int J Child Health Hum Dev 2018;11(1), in press.

[13] Hollenberg D, Ferguson T, Borean M, Anpalagan T, Rzepka A, Viehweger J, et al. Helmet use of young adults in Halifax, Canada. Int J Child Health Hum Dev 2018;11(1), in press.

[14] Chow R, Borean M, Murai A, Menon G, Hollenberg D, Anpalagan T, et al. Helmet use of young adults in California, United States of America. Int J Child Health Hum Dev 2018;11(1), in press.

[15] Chow R, Hollenberg D, Borean M, Goh S, Anpalagan T, Rzepka A, et al. Helmet use of young adults in Dublin, Ireland. Int J Child Health Hum Dev 2018;11(1), in press.

[16] Chow R, Hollenberg D, Pintilie A, Midroni C, Cumner S. Helmet use of adolescent cyclists at Crescent School in Toronto, Canada. Int J Adolesc Med Health 2016, in press

[17] Borean M, Ho S, Hollenberg D, Anpalagan T, Rzepka A, Viehweger J, et al. Helmet use of adolescents in Markham, Canada. Int J Adolesc Med Health 2017, in press.

[18] Borean M, Trasente V, Rzepka A, Viggiani D, Viotto D, Hollenberg D, et al. Helmet use of adolescents at De La Salle Oaklands in Toronto, Canada. Int J Child Health Hum Dev 2018;11(1), in press.

[19] Chow R, Borean M, Hollenberg D, Viehweger J, Young K, Young A, et al. Helmet use of adolescents at Ashbury College in Ottawa, Canada. Int J Child Health Hum Dev 2019, in press.

[20] Chow R, Borean M, Hollenberg D, Viehweger J, Hesse J. Helmet use of adolescents at Aberdeen Hall in Kelowna, Canada. Int J Child Health Hum Dev 2019, in press.

[21] Chow R, Borean M, Hollenberg D, Viehweger J, Alexander B, Gladstone J. Helmet use of adolescents at Linden School in Toronto, Canada. Int J Child Health Hum Dev 2019, in press.

[22] Viehweger J, Borean M, Hollenberg D, Cuzzetto S, Chow R. Helmet use of adolescents at Kamloops Christian School in Kamloops, Canada. Int J Child Health Hum Dev 2019, in press.

[23] Chow R, Borean M, Hollenberg D, Viehweger J, Smith B. Helmet use of adolescents at Southridge School in Surrey, Canada. Int J Child Health Hum Dev 2019, in press.

[24] Chow R, Borean M, Hollenberg D, Viehweger J. Helmet use of adolescents at Crestwood Preparatory College in Toronto, Canada. Int J Child Health Hum Dev 2019, in press.

[25] Chow R, Borean M, Hollenberg D, Viehweger J, Whitehouse J, Boughton C. Helmet use of adolescents at Elmwood School in Ottawa, Canada. Int J Child Health Hum Dev 2019, in press.

[26] Chow R, Viehweger J, Borean M, Hollenberg D. Helmet use of adolescents at Avon Old Farms School in Avon, USA. Int J Child Health Hum Dev 2019, in press.

[27] Anpalagan T, Borean M, Chen L, Viehweger J, Hollenberg D, Rzepka A, et al. Helmet use of adolescents in Toronto, Canada. Int J Child Health Hum Dev 2018;11(1), in press.

SECTION SIX: ACKNOWLEDGMENTS

In: Bicycles
Editors: Ronald Chow et al.

ISBN: 978-1-53612-458-3
© 2017 Nova Science Publishers, Inc.

Chapter 12

ABOUT THE EDITORS

Ronald Chow, BMSc(C), is the Founder and Chair of the Infinitas Research Group, headquartered in London, Ontario, Canada, and also the Founder and President of the Bicycle Safety and Awareness Club. At the young age of 19 years old, he already has over 140 peer-reviewed publications to his name. He was the recipient of the Ontario Lieutenant Governor's Community Volunteer Award for volunteerism in his community, the Chancellor's Scholarship from Queen's University for excellent academic ability and leadership skills, the George Eastman Young Leaders Award from the University of Rochester for astounding leadership and extensive extracurricular activities, and both the Future of Western Award and Innovation Award from the University of Western Ontario as the most accomplished first-year university student leader in the areas of academics, student government, athletics and philanthropy. Email: rchow48@uwo.ca

Michael Borean, BMSc(C), Deputy Chair of Infinitas Research Group and a Vice President of the Bicycle Safety and Awareness Club. He has a diverse research background. He has over 40 publications in peer-reviewed journals on topics including oncology, surgery, pharmacy, pediatrics, and public health. During his first year at Western University, Michael won the Innovation Award for leadership and extracurricular involvement. Outside of his research, Michael is heavily involved in student groups for health advocacy, student government, and athletics. He graduated from De La Salle College "Oaklands" in Toronto. Email: mborean@uwo.ca

Drew Hollenberg, BMSc(C), is a Deputy Chair of Infinitas Research Group and a Vice President of the Bicycle Safety and Awareness Club. Also, Drew has published over 50 papers in peer-reviewed journals at 19 years old. He was born in Canada, but soon moved to Tokyo, Japan and then to London, England. Finally returning to Canada again at the age of 14 years, Drew began high school at Crescent School where he won the Graduating Class trophy for outstanding service to the school. Now at Western University, Drew is studying a bachelor in medical sciences. Email: dhollen@uwo.ca

Jaclyn Viehweger, BMSc(C), is the Secretary of the Bicyle Safety and Awareness Club. Jaclyn is also a Varsity Cheerleader with the University of Western Ontario Mustangs. She holds the Gold Duke of Edinburgh Award for her service in the community and commitment to extracurriculars and athletics. Jaclyn graduated from Holy Name of Mary College School in Mississauga having received the Sister Celestine Giertych Social Justice Award and is now at Western University pursuing a Bachelor of Medical Sciences. Email: jviehweg@uwo.ca

Tharani Anpalagan, BMSc(C), is a proud member of Infinitas Research Group and a Vice President of the Bicycle Safety and Awareness Club. Tharani was the recipient of the Western National President's Scholarship for excellence in academics and extracuricular activities and the National Future Aces Scholarship for her community service. Upon graduation from her high school, she also received the Character Education Award. Tharani is now studying at Western University in the Medical Sciences program. She won the innovation award in first year for her leadership and extracurricular involvement. Email: tanpalag@uwo.ca

Anna Rzepka, BMSc(C), is a Vice President of the Bicycle Safety and Awareness Club and a founding researcher for the Infinitas Research Group. Anna was the recipient of the Governor General's Academic Medal for the highest graduating average in her secondary school, and has won the Innovation Award for leadership during her first year at Western University. Anna remains highly involved charitable organizations, the university choir, and operating her online business which she founded in 2014. Email: arzepka@uwo.ca

Joav Merrick, MD, MMedSci, DMSc, born and educated in Denmark is professor of pediatrics, child health and human development, Division of Pediatrics, Hadassah Hebrew University Medical Center, Mt Scopus Campus, Jerusalem, Israel and Kentucky Children's Hospital, University of Kentucky, Lexington, Kentucky United States and professor of public health at the Center for Healthy Development, School of Public Health, Georgia State University, Atlanta, United States, the medical director of the Health Services, Division for Intellectual and Developmental Disabilities, Ministry of Social Affairs and Social Services, Jerusalem, the founder and director of the National Institute of Child Health and Human Development in Israel. Numerous publications in the field of pediatrics, child health and human development, rehabilitation, intellectual disability, disability, health, welfare, abuse, advocacy, quality of life and prevention. Received the Peter Sabroe Child Award for outstanding work on behalf of Danish Children in 1985 and the International LEGO-Prize ("The Children's Nobel Prize") for an extraordinary contribution towards improvement in child welfare and well-being in 1987. Email: jmerrick@zahav.net.il

In: Bicycles
Editors: Ronald Chow et al.

ISBN: 978-1-53612-458-3
© 2017 Nova Science Publishers, Inc.

Chapter 13

ABOUT INFINITAS RESEARCH GROUP, LONDON, ONTARIO, CANADA

Infinitas Research Group (IRG) was founded in 2017, and is currently headquartered in London, Ontario, Canada. Research associates are based around the globe (across Canada, United States, Europe, Asia and Australia), allowing for IRG to conduct research studies on an international scale.

IRG has a special interest in public health issues, and specializes into studying the adolescent and young adult population. Thus far, IRG members have worked in collaboration with the Bicycle Safety and Awareness Club in London, Canada, to investigate bicycle safety practices of adolescents and young adults and a project to investigate adolescent and youg adult awareness about Alzheimer's disease in partnership with the Alzheimer's Western Club of the University of Western Ontario (London, Ontario, Canada).

Contact
Ronald Chow
Founder and Chair,
Infinitas Research Group,
London, Ontario, Canada
Email: rchow48@uwo.ca

In: Bicycles
Editors: Ronald Chow et al.

ISBN: 978-1-53612-458-3
© 2017 Nova Science Publishers, Inc.

Chapter 14

ABOUT THE BICYCLE SAFETY AND AWARENESS CLUB, LONDON, ONTARIO, CANADA

The Bicycle Safety and Awareness Club (BSAC) is a student-run organization headquartered in London, Ontario, Canada. It was established in 2016, and has affiliated members located in Canada, United States and other countries. The aim of BSAC is to educate, advocate and promote bicycle safety among university students and the young adult population in the local community. Advocating and educating about safe cycling practices are centrally-managed by the operations team at headquarters in London, Canada.

The research arm of BSAC operates independently of the operations team. It draws on resources available to BSAC as needed to investigate and evaluate current cycling practices in communities. This present book, for example, is a culmination of the research work conducted by BSAC's research team.

With the knowledge uncovered by the research arm, the operations team acts accordingly to cater its advocacy/education programs towards the local communities. BSAC coordinately works towards building a safer and better community for student and young adult cyclists.

Contact

Ronald Chow
Founder and President,
Bicycle Safety and Awareness Club,
London, Ontario, Canada
Email: rchow48@uwo.ca

In: Bicycles
Editors: Ronald Chow et al.
ISBN: 978-1-53612-458-3
© 2017 Nova Science Publishers, Inc.

Chapter 15

ABOUT THE NATIONAL INSTITUTE OF CHILD HEALTH AND HUMAN DEVELOPMENT IN ISRAEL

The National Institute of Child Health and Human Development (NICHD) in Israel was established in 1998 as a virtual institute under the auspices of the Medical Director, Ministry of Social Affairs and Social Services in order to function as the research arm for the Office of the Medical Director. In 1998 the National Council for Child Health and Pediatrics, Ministry of Health and in 1999 the Director General and Deputy Director General of the Ministry of Health endorsed the establishment of the NICHD.

Mission

The mission of a National Institute for Child Health and Human Development in Israel is to provide an academic focal point for the scholarly interdisciplinary study of child life, health, public health, welfare, disability, rehabilitation, intellectual disability and related aspects of human development. This mission includes research, teaching, clinical work, information and public service activities in the field of child health and human development.

Service and academic activities

Over the years many activities became focused in the south of Israel due to collaboration with various professionals at the Faculty of Health Sciences (FOHS) at the Ben Gurion University of the Negev (BGU). Since 2000 an affiliation with the Zusman Child Development Center at the Pediatric Division of Soroka University Medical Center has resulted in collaboration around the establishment of the Down Syndrome Clinic at that center. In 2002 a full course on "Disability" was established at the Recanati School for Allied Professions in the Community, FOHS, BGU and in 2005 collaboration was started with the Primary Care Unit of the faculty and disability became part of the master of public health course on "Children and society". In the academic year 2005-2006 a one semester course on "Aging with disability" was started as part of the master of science program in gerontology in our collaboration with the Center for Multidisciplinary Research in Aging. In 2010 collaborations with the Division of Pediatrics, Hadassah Hebrew University Medical Center, Jerusalem, Israel around the National Down Syndrome Center and teaching students and residents about intellectual and developmental disabilities as part of their training at this campus.

Research activities

The affiliated staff have over the years published work from projects and research activities in this national and international collaboration. In the year 2000 the International Journal of Adolescent Medicine and

Health and in 2005 the International Journal on Disability and Human Development of De Gruyter Publishing House (Berlin and New York) were affiliated with the National Institute of Child Health and Human Development. From 2008 also the International Journal of Child Health and Human Development (Nova Science, New York), the International Journal of Child and Adolescent Health (Nova Science) and the Journal of Pain Management (Nova Science) affiliated and from 2009 the International Public Health Journal (Nova Science) and Journal of Alternative Medicine Research (Nova Science). All peer-reviewed international journals.

National collaborations

Nationally the NICHD works in collaboration with the Faculty of Health Sciences, Ben Gurion University of the Negev; Department of Physical Therapy, Sackler School of Medicine, Tel Aviv University; Autism Center, Assaf HaRofeh Medical Center; National Rett and PKU Centers at Chaim Sheba Medical Center, Tel HaShomer; Department of Physiotherapy, Haifa University; Department of Education, Bar Ilan University, Ramat Gan, Faculty of Social Sciences and Health Sciences; College of Judea and Samaria in Ariel and in 2011 affiliation with Center for Pediatric Chronic Diseases and National Center for Down Syndrome, Department of Pediatrics, Hadassah Hebrew University Medical Center, Mount Scopus Campus, Jerusalem.

International collaborations

Internationally with the Department of Disability and Human Development, College of Applied Health Sciences, University of Illinois at Chicago; Strong Center for Developmental Disabilities,

Golisano Children's Hospital at Strong, University of Rochester School of Medicine and Dentistry, New York; Centre on Intellectual Disabilities, University of Albany, New York; Centre for Chronic Disease Prevention and Control, Health Canada, Ottawa; Chandler Medical Center and Children's Hospital, Kentucky Children's Hospital, Section of Adolescent Medicine, University of Kentucky, Lexington; Chronic Disease Prevention and Control Research Center, Baylor College of Medicine, Houston, Texas; Division of Neuroscience, Department of Psychiatry, Columbia University, New York; Institute for the Study of Disadvantage and Disability, Atlanta; Center for Autism and Related Disorders, Department Psychiatry, Children's Hospital Boston, Boston; Department of Pediatric and Adolescent Medicine, Western Michigan University Homer Stryker MD School of Medicine, Kalamazoo, Michigan, United States; Department of Paediatrics, Child Health and Adolescent Medicine, Children's Hospital at Westmead, Westmead, Australia; International Centre for the Study of Occupational and Mental Health, Düsseldorf, Germany; Centre for Advanced Studies in Nursing, Department of General Practice and Primary Care, University of Aberdeen, Aberdeen, United Kingdom; Quality of Life Research Center, Copenhagen, Denmark; Nordic School of Public Health, Gottenburg, Sweden, Scandinavian Institute of Quality of Working Life, Oslo, Norway; The Department of Applied Social Sciences (APSS) of The Hong Kong Polytechnic University Hong Kong.

Targets

Our focus is on research, international collaborations, clinical work, teaching and policy in health, disability and human development and to establish the NICHD as a permanent institute in Israel in order to conduct model research and together with the four university schools of public health/medicine in Israel establish a national master and doctoral program in disability and human development at the institute to secure the next generation of professionals working in this often non-prestigious/low-status field of work.

Contact

Joav Merrick, MD, MMedSci, DMSc
Professor of Pediatrics
Medical Director, Health Services, Division for Intellectual and Developmental Disabilities, Ministry of Social Affairs and Social Services, POB 1260, IL-91012 Jerusalem, Israel.
E-mail: jmerrick@zahav.net.il

In: Bicycles
Editors: Ronald Chow et al.

ISBN: 978-1-53612-458-3
© 2017 Nova Science Publishers, Inc.

Chapter 16

ABOUT THE BOOK SERIES "PEDIATRICS, CHILD AND ADOLESCENT HEALTH"

Pediatrics, child and adolescent health is a book series with publications from a multidisciplinary group of researchers, practitioners and clinicians for an international professional forum interested in the broad spectrum of pediatric medicine, child health, adolescent health and human development.

- Merrick J, ed. Child and adolescent health yearbook 2011. New York: Nova Science, 2012.
- Merrick J, ed. Child and adolescent health yearbook 2012. New York: Nova Science, 2012.
- Roach RR, Greydanus DE, Patel DR, Homnick DN, Merrick J, eds. Tropical pediatrics: A public health concern of international proportions. New York: Nova Science, 2012.
- Merrick J, ed. Child health and human development yearbook 2011. New York: Nova Science, 2012.
- Merrick J, ed. Child health and human development yearbook 2012. New York: Nova Science, 2012.
- Shek DTL, Sun RCF, Merrick J, eds. Developmental issues in Chinese adolescents. New York: Nova Science, 2012.

- Shek DTL, Sun RCF, Merrick J, eds. Positive youth development: Theory, research and application. New York: Nova Science, 2012.
- Zachor DA, Merrick J, eds. Understanding autism spectrum disorder: Current research aspects. New York: Nova Science, 2012.
- Ma HK, Shek DTL, Merrick J, eds. Positive youth development: A new school curriculum to tackle adolescent developmental issues. New York: Nova Science, 2012.
- Wood D, Reiss JG, Ferris ME, Edwards LR, Merrick J, eds. Transition from pediatric to adult medical care. New York: Nova Science, 2012.
- Isenberg Y. Guidelines for the healthy integration of the ill child in the educational system: Experience from Israel. New York: Nova Science, 2013.
- Shek DTL, Sun RCF, Merrick J, eds. Chinese adolescent development: Economic disadvantages, parents and intrapersonal development. New York: Nova Science, 2013.
- Shek DTL, Sun RCF, Merrick J, eds. University and college students: Health and development issues for the leaders of tomorrow. New York: Nova Science, 2013.
- Shek DTL, Sun RCF, Merrick J, eds. Adolescence and behavior issues in a Chinese context. New York: Nova Science, 2013.
- Sun J, Buys N, Merrick J. Advances in preterm infant research. New York: Nova Science, 2013.
- Tsitsika A, Janikian M, Greydanus DE, Omar HA, Merrick J, eds. Internet addiction: A public health concern in adolescence. New York: Nova Science, 2013.
- Shek, DTL, Lee TY, Merrick J, eds. Promotion of holistic development of young people in Hong Kong. New York: Nova Science, 2013.
- Shek DTL, Ma C, Lu Y, Merrick J, eds. Human developmental research: Experience from research in Hong Kong. New York: Nova Science, 2013.
- Rubin IL, Merrick J, eds. Child health and human development: Social, economic and environmental factors. New York: Nova Science, 2013.

- Merrick J, ed. Chronic disease and disability in childhood. New York: Nova Science, 2013.
- Rubin IL, Merrick J, eds. Break the cycle of environmental health disparities: Maternal and child health aspects. New York: Nova Science, 2013.
- Rubin IL, Merrick J, eds. Environmental health disparities in children: Asthma, obesity and food. New York: Nova Science, 2013.
- Rubin IL, Merrick J, eds. Environmental health: Home, school and community. New York: Nova Science, 2013.
- Merrick J, Kandel I, Omar HA, eds. Children, violence and bullying: International perspectives. New York: Nova Science, 2013.
- Omar HA, Bowling CH, Merrick J, eds. Playing with fire: Children, adolescents and firesetting. New York: Nova Science, 2013.
- Merrick J, Tenenbaum A, Omar HA, eds. School, adolescence and health issues. New York: Nova Science, 2014.
- Merrick J, Tenenbaum A, Omar HA, eds. Adolescence and sexuality: International perspectives. New York: Nova Science, 2014.
- Diamond G, Arbel E. Adoption: The search for a new parenthood adoption. New York: Nova Science, 2014.
- Taylor MF, Pooley JA, Merrick J, eds. Adolescence: Places and spaces. New York: Nova Science, 2014.
- Greydanus DE, Feinberg AN, Merrick J, eds. Born into this world: Health issues. New York: Nova Science, 2014.
- Greydanus DE, Feinberg AN, Merrick J, eds. Caring for the newborn: A comprehensive guide for the clinician. New York: Nova Science, 2014.
- Rubin IL, Merrick J, eds. Environment and hope: Improving health, reducing AIDS and promoting food security in the world. New York: Nova Science, 2014.
- Greydanus DE, Feinberg AN, Merrick J, eds. Pediatric and adolescent dermatology: Some current issues. New York: Nova Science, 2014.

- Roach RR, Greydanus DE, Patel DR, Merrick J, eds. Tropical pediatrics: A public helath concern of international proportions, Second edition. New York: Nova Science, 2015.
- Merrick J, ed. Child and adolescent health issues: A tribute to the pediatrician Donald E Greydanus. New York: Nova Science, 2015.
- Feinberg AN. A pediatric resident pocket guide: Making the most of morning reports. New York: Nova Science, 2015.
- Greydanus DE, Patel DR, Pratt HD, Calles Jr JL, Nazeer A, Merrick J, eds. Behavioral pediatrics, 4th edition. New York: Nova Science, 2015.
- Merrick J, ed. Disability, chronic disease and human development. New York: Nova Science, 2015.
- Hegamin-Younger C, Merrick J, eds. Caribbean adolescents: Some public health concerns. New York: Nova Science, 2015.
- Merrick J, ed. Adolescence and health: Some international perspectives. New York: Nova Science, 2015.
- Omar HA. Youth suicide prevention: Everybody's business. New York: Nova Science, 2015.
- Greydanus DE, Raj VMS, Merrick J, eds. Chronic disease and disability: The pediatric kidney. New York: Nova Science, 2015.
- Merrick J, ed. Children and childhood: Some international aspects. New York: Nova Science, 2016.
- Shek DTL, Lee TY, Merrick J, eds. Children and adolescents: Future challenges. New York: Nova Science, 2016.
- Shek DTL, Wu FKU, Leung JTY, Merrick J, eds. Adolescence: Positive youth development programs in Chinese communities. New York: Nova Science, 2016.
- Merrick J, Greydanus DE, eds. Sexuality: Some international aspects. New York: Nova Science, 2016.
- Harel-Fisch Y, Abdeen Z, Navot M. Growing up in the Middle East: The daily lives and well-being of Israeli and Palestinian youth. New York: Nova Science, 2016.
- Greydanus DE, Malhotra D, Merrick J, eds. Chronic disease and disability: The pediatric heart. New York: Nova Science, 2016.

- Greydanus DE, Kamboj MK, Merrick J, eds. Chronic disease and disability: The pediatric pancreas. New York: Nova Science, 2016.
- Kamboj MK, Greydanus DE, Merrick J, eds. Diabetes mellitus: Childhood and adolescence. New York: Nova Science, 2016.
- Greydanus DE, Palusci VJ, Merrick J, eds. Chronic disease and disability: Abuse and neglect in childhood and adolescence. New York: Nova Science, 2016.
- Greydanus DE, Calles JL Jr, Patel DR, Nazeer A, Merrick J, eds. Clinical aspects of psychopharmacology in childhood and adlescence, second ed. New York: Nova Science, 2016.
- Greydanus DE, Apple RW, White K, Merrick J, eds. Children and youth: Post-traumatic stress disorder and motor vehicle crashes. New York: Nova Science, 2017.
- Mazaba ML, Siziya S, Merrick J, eds. Suicide: A global view on suicidal ideation among adolescents. New York: Nova Science, 2017.
- Chow R, Merrick J, eds. Adolescence: Bicycle and helmet use of adolescents and young adults. New York: Nova Science, 2017.

Contact

Professor Joav Merrick, MD, MMedSci, DMSc
Medical Director, Medical Services
Division for Intellectual and Developmental Disabilities
Ministry of Social Affairs and Social Services
POBox 1260, IL-91012 Jerusalem, Israel
E-mail: jmerrick@zahav.net.il

SECTION SEVEN: INDEX

INDEX

A

Aberdeen Hall, 29, 39, 49, 53, 55, 67, 69, 78, 89, 108
abuse, 113
adolescent boys, 16, 21, 62, 71, 72, 94
adolescent development, 58, 126
adolescents, 3, 4, 5, 6, 7, 8, 15, 16, 17, 22, 23, 25, 27, 28, 29, 31, 32, 37, 38, 39, 40, 41, 42, 49, 53, 54, 58, 60, 61, 62, 67, 68, 69, 70, 71, 72, 77, 78, 81, 82, 87, 88, 89, 93, 94, 95, 96, 97, 98, 99, 101, 103, 104, 105, 106, 107, 108, 115, 125, 127, 128, 129
adults, 4, 16, 54, 62, 94
advocacy, 112, 113, 117
age, 4, 16, 19, 20, 21, 23, 24, 25, 26, 27, 28, 32, 37, 38, 41, 42, 44, 47, 54, 58, 59, 61, 62, 64, 67, 68, 72, 74, 76, 77, 82, 86, 87, 93, 94, 95, 105, 106, 111, 112
Ashbury College, 15, 16, 17, 21, 29, 39, 49, 60, 69, 78, 89, 108
Asia, 115
autism, 126
Avon, 40, 49, 70, 81, 82, 83, 108
Avon Old Farms School, 40, 49, 70, 81, 83, 108
awareness, 18, 20, 28, 32, 37, 38, 67, 82, 87, 88, 115

B

benefits, 21, 42, 47, 67, 72, 76, 77, 82, 87, 88
bias, 21, 28, 37, 47, 59, 67, 77, 87
bicycle, 3, 4, 5, 7, 8, 9, 11, 15, 16, 17, 22, 23, 25, 29, 31, 32, 33, 37, 39, 40, 41, 42, 43, 44, 49, 53, 55, 57, 60, 61, 63, 68, 70, 71, 72, 73, 76, 77, 78, 81, 82, 83, 86, 87, 89, 93, 94, 95, 96, 97, 98, 99, 101, 103, 104, 105, 106, 107, 111, 112,113, 115, 117, 118, 129
British Columbia, 51, 53, 55, 59, 61, 62, 68, 71, 72, 73, 82
bullying, 127

C

Canada, 3, 4, 5, 6, 7, 15, 16, 17, 22, 23, 24, 25, 29, 31, 32, 33, 38, 39, 40, 41, 42, 43,

Index

48, 49, 53, 54, 55, 59, 60, 61, 62, 63, 68, 69, 71, 72, 73, 77, 78, 81, 82, 88, 89, 93, 94, 107, 108, 111, 112, 115, 116, 117, 118, 122
Caribbean, 128
causation, 16, 21
challenges, 128
charitable organizations, 113
Chicago, 121
childhood, 58, 67, 87, 127, 128, 129
children, 47, 127
collaboration, 4, 115, 120, 121
college students, **126**
communities, 117, 118, 128
community, 111, 112, 118, 127
community service, 113
correlation, 4, 5, 16, 21, 23, 24, 26, 28, 32, 37, 38, 41, 47, 54, 58, 59, 62, 67, 68, 71, 72, 77, 82, 87, 88, 93, 105, 106
Crestwood Preparatory College, 31, 33, 108
cycling, 9, 19, 20, 27, 35, 36, 46, 53, 54, 59, 66, 67, 76, 82, 85, 87, 88, 117

D

Denmark, 113, 122
Department of Education, 121
detection, 5, 16, 28
deviation, 82, 88
diabetes, 129
disability, 113, 119, 120, 122, 127, 128, 129
disorder, 126, 129

E

education, 28, 65, 87, 117
educational programs, 32, 37, 38, 67, 72, 76, 77
educational system, 126
encouragement, 16, 21, 22, 37, 54, 59, 62, 67, 68

England, 112
environment, 23, 24, 28, 58, 67, 77, 82, 87, 88
environmental factors, 58, 67, 126
equipment, 37
Europe, 115

G

geography, 72
Georgia, 4, 113
Germany, 122
gerontology, 120
grades, 17, 33, 43, 55, 61, 63, 83

H

head injury(ies), 28, 94
head trauma, 61, 62, 94
health, 58, 112, 113, 119, 122, 125, 126, 127, 128
helmet use, 3, 4, 5, 6, 7, 8, 9, 11, 15, 16, 17, 18, 19, 20, 21, 22, 23, 24, 25, 26, 27, 28, 29, 31, 32, 33, 34, 35, 37, 38, 39, 40, 41, 42, 43, 44, 45, 46, 47, 48, 49, 53, 54, 55, 56, 57, 58, 59, 60, 61, 62, 63, 64, 65, 67, 68, 69, 70, 71, 72, 73, 74, 75, 77, 78, 81, 82, 83, 84, 85, 86, 87, 88, 89, 93, 94, 95, 96, 97, 98, 99, 101, 103, 104, 105, 106, 107, 108, 129
high school, 5, 24, 72, 73, 95, 112, 113
Hong Kong, 122, 126
human, 28, 113, 120, 122, 125, 126, 128
human development, 113, 120, 122, 125, 126, 128

I

individuals, 4, 8, 16, 21, 25, 28, 32, 34, 37, 38, 54, 67, 72, 77

Index

injury(ies), 4, 28
integration, 126
Ireland, 6, 39, 49, 69, 107
Israel, 3, 113, 119, 120, 122, 123, 126, 129
issues, 115, 125, 126, 127, 128

J

Japan, 112

K

Kamloops, 40, 49, 69, 71, 89, 108
Kamloops Christian School, 40, 49, 69, 89, 108
Kelowna, 29, 39, 49, 53, 55, 59, 69, 78, 89, 108

L

law enforcement, 32, 37, 38
leadership, 111, 112, 113
legislation, 8, 9, 17, 18, 19, 20, 25, 26, 27, 28, 32, 33, 34, 35, 37, 38, 42, 43, 44, 47, 54, 55, 56, 57, 58, 63, 64, 65, 67, 72, 73, 74, 76, 77, 82, 83, 84, 86, 87, 88, 94, 95, 103, 104, 106
Linden School, 23, 24, 25, 40, 49, 69, 78, 89, 108
local community, 117

M

majority, 16, 18, 19, 21, 22, 44, 45, 57, 64, 74, 84
media, 21, 87
medical, 112, 113, 126
medical care, 126
medical science, 112
medicine, 123, 125

mellitus, 129
meta-analysis, 4, 5, 15, 16, 17, 21, 22, 24, 29, 32, 39, 42, 49, 54, 60, 61, 62, 68, 72, 77, 82, 89, 93, 94, 95, 104, 106, 107
Middle East, 128
mission, 119
multiple-choice questions, 11

N

neglect, 129
next generation, 123
Nobel Prize, 113
North America, 4, 95, 102, 104, 105
Norway, 122

O

obesity, 127
operations, 117
Ottawa, 15, 17, 29, 39, 41, 42, 43, 49, 53, 54, 60, 69, 78, 89, 108, 122

P

pancreas, 129
parental influence, 77
parenthood, 127
parents, 126
participants, 8, 73
pediatrician, 128
policy, 122
population, 5, 15, 16, 24, 27, 28, 32, 37, 38, 47, 54, 59, 62, 67, 76, 87, 94, 106, 115, 117
positive correlation, 32, 42, 94
preparation, 106
president, 111, 112, 118
prevention, 113, 128
professionals, 120, 123

project, 115
psychopharmacology, 129
public health, 112, 113, 115, 119, 120, 123, 125, 126, 128
public schools, 95, 104
public service, 120

Q

quality of life, 113
questionnaire, 7, 8, 16, 17, 22, 24, 25, 29, 31, 33, 38, 42, 43, 48, 54, 55, 56, 59, 61, 62, 63, 68, 72, 73, 74, 77, 81, 83, 88

R

reasoning, 17, 25, 33, 42, 43, 54, 55, 63, 73, 81, 83
recreational, 5, 9, 11, 17, 19, 20, 21, 25, 26, 27, 33, 35, 36, 37, 42, 43, 44, 45, 46, 47, 55, 57, 58, 59, 63, 65, 66, 67, 72, 73, 74, 75, 76, 83, 85, 86, 94, 95, 97, 99, 103, 104, 105, 106
recruiting, 67
rehabilitation, 113, 119
researchers, 125
resources, 117
response, 21, 28, 37, 47, 54, 59, 67, 77, 87

S

safety, 7, 16, 17, 37, 42, 47, 54, 58, 67, 82, 87, 88, 94, 95, 115, 117
SAS, 18, 25, 33, 43, 55, 63, 73, 83
school, 4, 5, 7, 8, 11, 16, 17, 18, 19, 21, 23, 24, 25, 26, 27, 28, 31, 32, 33, 34, 36, 42, 43, 44, 45, 46, 47, 53, 54, 55, 56, 57, 58, 61, 62, 63, 64, 66, 67, 71, 72, 73, 74, 75, 76, 81, 82, 83, 84, 85, 86, 87, 88, 94, 95, 96, 98, 101, 103, 104, 105, 106, 112, 113, 122, 126, 127
science, 120
secondary schools, 53, 54
society, 120
Southridge School, 40, 49, 61, 62, 108
statistics, 11, 17, 25, 33, 43, 55, 63, 73, 83
stress, 129
student populations, 72
subgroups, 73
suicidal ideation, 129
suicide, 128
Sun, 125, 126
Surrey, 40, 49, 61, 62, 68, 108
survey instrument, xv, 7, 22, 29, 40, 49, 60, 70, 78, 89
Sweden, 122

T

Toronto, 4, 6, 15, 16, 17, 22, 23, 24, 25, 29, 31, 32, 33, 39, 40, 48, 49, 53, 54, 60, 68, 69, 77, 78, 82, 88, 89, 94, 107, 108, 112
training, 120
transportation, 17, 25, 33, 42, 43, 47, 55, 63, 72, 73, 83
trauma, 28

U

United Kingdom, 122
United States (USA), 4, 5, 6, 38, 39, 40, 48, 49, 68, 69, 70, 79, 81, 81, 83, 87, 88, 107, 108, 113, 115, 117, 122

V

variations, 5
Vice President, 111, 112, 113
violence, 127

volunteerism, 111

W

wear, 8, 16, 17, 18, 20, 25, 27, 32, 33, 36, 37, 38, 41, 43, 53, 55, 56, 57, 63, 65, 67, 72, 73, 74, 81, 82, 83
welfare, 113, 119
well-being, 58, 113, 128
workload, 37
worry, 20

Y

yield, 17, 25, 33, 43, 55, 63, 73, 83
young adults, 4, 5, 6, 7, 16, 22, 29, 32, 38, 39, 42, 48, 49, 54, 60, 62, 68, 69, 77, 89, 94, 95, 107, 115, 129
young people, 126